Chinese Medicine

Modern Practice

Annals of Traditional Chinese Medicine – Vol. 1

Chinese Medicine

Modern Practice

editors

Ping-chung Leung
The Chinese University of Hong Kong

Charlie Chang-li Xue
RMIT University, Australia

World Scientific

NEW JERSEY • LONDON • SINGAPORE • BEIJING • SHANGHAI • HONG KONG • TAIPEI • CHENNAI

Published by

World Scientific Publishing Co. Pte. Ltd.
5 Toh Tuck Link, Singapore 596224
USA office: 27 Warren Street, Suite 401-402, Hackensack, NJ 07601
UK office: 57 Shelton Street, Covent Garden, London WC2H 9HE

British Library Cataloguing-in-Publication Data
A catalogue record for this book is available from the British Library.

CHINESE MEDICINE — MODERN PRACTICE

ISBN 981-256-018-1

Printed in Singapore by World Scientific Printers (S) Pte Ltd

Contents

Contributors

Kelvin Chan
School of Chinese Medicine
Hong Kong Baptist University
Hong Kong, China

Chang Chen
Tianjin Institute of Acute Abdominal Diseases by Integrated Medicine
Tianjin, China

Ke-ji Chen
Xi-yuan Hospital
China Academy of Traditional Chinese Medicine
Beijing, China

Zhi-shan Ding
Research Institute of Molecular Medicine
Zhejiang College of Traditional Chinese Medicine
Hongzhou, China

Edzard Ernst
Peninsula Medical School
University of Exeter & Plymouth
Exeter, UK

Ji-qian Fang
School of Public Health
Sun Yat-Sen University
Guangzhou, China

Chong-fen Guan
Institute of Basic Theory of Traditional Chinese Medicine
China Academy of Traditional Chinese Medicine
Beijing, China

Yi-yang Hu
Shanghai University of Traditional Chinese Medicine
Shanghai, China

Pei-xin Huang
Guang Dong Provincial Hospital of TCM
Guangdong, China

Yan Huang
Guang Dong Provincial Hospital of TCM
Guangdong, China

Wei Jia
Xi-yuan Hospital
National Research Institute of Traditional Chinese Medicine
Beijing, China

Kwok-fai Leung
Department of Occupational Therapy
Queen Elizabeth Hospital
Hong Kong, China

Ping-chung Leung
Institute of Chinese Medicine
The Chinese University of Hong Kong
Hong Kong, China

Jun Li
Chongzhou Demobilized Soldier Hospital
Sichuan, China

Jian-hua Lin
Acupuncture and Moxibustion College
Chengdu University of Traditional Chinese Medicine
Sichuan, China

Robyn Lines
Program Renewal
Royal Melbourne Institute of Technology
Victoria, Australia

Cheng Liu
Shanghai University of Traditional Chinese Medicine
Shanghai, China

Cheng-hai Liu
Shanghai University of Traditional Chinese Medicine
Shanghai, China

Feng-bin Liu
The First Affiliated Hospital
Guangzhou University of Traditional Chinese Medicine
Guangzhou, China

Jia-xiang Liu
Longhua Hospital Affiliated to Shanghai University of Traditional Chinese Medicine
Shanghai, China

Mao-cai Liu
Guangdong Provincial Hospital of Traditional Chinese Medicine
TWGHs Kwong Wah Hospital — Chinese Medicine Clinical Research and Services Centre
The Chinese University of Hong Kong
Hong Kong, China

Ping Liu
Shanghai University of Traditional Chinese Medicine
Shanghai, China

Ming Lu
Guang Dong Provincial Hospital of TCM
Guangdong, China

Wei-bo Lu
China Academy of Traditional Chinese Medicine
Beijing, China

Yong-fen Luo
Acupuncture and Moxibustion College
Chengdu University of Traditional Chinese Medicine
Chongzhou Demobilized Soldier Hospital
Sichuan, China

Xiao-chang Ma
Xi-yuan Hospital
China Academy of Traditional Chinese Medicine
Beijing, China

Kylie A. O'Brien
Division of Chinese Medicine
Royal Melbourne Institute of Technology
Victoria, Australia

Da-zhuo Shi
Xi-yuan Hospital
China Academy of Traditional Chinese Medicine
Beijing, China

Zai-shan Tian
Tianjin Institute of Acute Abdominal Diseases by Integrated Medicine
Tianjin, China

Jie Wang
Xi-yuan Hospital
National Research Institute of Traditional Chinese Medicine
Beijing, China

Eric Wong
Nikyang Enterprise Ltd. Co.
Hong Kong

Gen-cheng Wu
Institute of Acupuncture Research
WHO Collaborating Centre for Traditional Medicine
Shanghai Medical College, Fudan University
Shanghai, China

Jun-mei Wu
Acupuncture and Moxibustion College
Chengdu University of Traditional Chinese Medicine
Sichuan, China

Xian-zhong Wu
Tianjin Institute of Acute Abdominal Diseases by Integrated Medicine
Tianjin, China

Pei-shan Xie
Guangzhou Institute for Drug Control
Guangdong, China

Hao Xu
Xi-yuan Hospital
China Academy of Traditional Chinese Medicine
Beijing, China

Lie-ming Xu
Shanghai University of Traditional Chinese Medicine
Shanghai, China

Charlie Chang-li Xue
The Chinese Medicine Unit
Royal Melbourne Institute of Technology
Victoria, Australia

Xing-de Yuo
Research Institute of Molecular Medicine
Zhejiang College of Traditional Chinese Medicine
Hongzhou, China

Lin-guo Zhang
Xi-yuan Hospital
National Research Institute of Traditional Chinese Medicine
Beijing, China

Li Zhao
School of Chinese Medicine
Hong Kong Baptist University
Hong Kong, China

Preface to Series

Does Traditional Chinese Medicine Work?

History should be acknowledged and respected. Despite this, the historical value of Chinese medicine in China and some parts of Asia should not be used as the only important evidence of efficacy.

While clinical science has followed closely the principles of deductive research in science and developed its methodology of wide acceptance, there is a natural demand from both users and service providers that the same methodology be applied to the traditional art of healing. There should be only one scale for the measurement of efficacy. Thus, evidence-based medicine, which apparently is the only acceptable form of treatment, would also claim its sovereignty in Chinese medicine.

In spite of influential proponents and diligent practitioners, efforts relating to the application of evidence-based medicine methodology to Chinese medicine research have been slow and unimpressive. This should not come as a surprise. Evidence-based medicine requires the knowledge of the exact chemistry of the drug used, the exact physical or chemical activities involved and above all, the biological responses in the recipient. All these are not known. Working back from the black box of old historical records of efficacy requires huge resources and time, if at all possible. Insistence on this approach would result in either unending frustrations or utter desperation.

Parallel with the modern attempts, respectable Chinese medicine practitioners have unendingly and relentlessly cried out their objection to the evidence-based approach. They insisted that all the evidences were already there from the Classical Records. Forcing the classical applications through a rigid modern framework of scrutiny is artificially coating Chinese medicine with a scientific clothing that does not fit.

Thus, the modern proponents are facing an impasse when they rely totally on modern scientific concepts. The traditional converts are persisting to push their pilgrims of defense. Where do we stand so as to achieve the best results of harmonisation?

There must be a compromise somewhere. Classic evidences can be transformed into a universal language to be fairly evaluated and to be decided whether suitable for further research, using the deductive methodology or an innovative one after intelligent modifications.

There is a need for a platform on which a direction can be developed in the attempt to modernise the traditional art and science of healing, while remaining free and objective to utilise the decaying wisdom without prejudice.

With the growing demand for complementary/alternative medicine from the global public and a parallel interest from the service providers, there is an urgent need for the provision of valuable information in this area.

The Annals of Chinese Medicine is a timely serial publication responding to this need. It will be providing authoritative and current information about Chinese medicine in the areas of clinical trials, biological activities of herbs, education, research and quality control requirements. Contributors are invited to send in their reports and reviews to ensure quality and value. Clinicians and scientists who are willing to submit their valuable observations, resulting from their painstaking researches are welcome to send in their manuscripts. *The Annals of Chinese Medicine* has the objective of providing a lasting platform for all who concentrate their efforts on the modernization of Chinese medicine.

Professor Ping-chung Leung
Institute of Chinese Medicine
The Chinese University of Hong Kong

Chapter 1

Risks of Traditional Chinese Herbal Medicine

Edzard Ernst

Abstract

The popularity of Traditional Chinese Herbal Medicine (TCHM) is considerable and increasing. It is therefore important to be aware of its risks. These mainly relate to the toxicity of some herbal ingredients, to the contamination/adulteration of some products and to herb-drug interactions. Rather than providing an exhaustive review of these complex subjects, examples are provided for each of these categories. They demonstrate that TCHMs are not devoid of risks. The size of the problem is, however, difficult to identify — quite simply, our present knowledge is too incomplete. It follows that, in the interest of consumers' safety, the systematic study of this area should be encouraged.

Keywords: Herbal Medicine; Risks; Toxicity; Interactions.

1.1 Introduction

During the last two decades, Traditional Chinese Herbal Medicines (TCHMs) have increasingly fascinated consumers, health care providers and researchers in the West. It has been estimated that 300,000 practitioners of TCHM practise in over 140 countries worldwide (Scheid, 2000). This stunning success of TCHM has prompted some enthusiasts to speak of the 21st century as "the century of TCHM".

Given its increasing popularity, it is timely and necessary to review the risks that have been associated with the use of TCHMs. They may be linked mainly to the toxicity of some herbal ingredients, to the effects of contaminants/adulterants or to herb-drug interactions. Because

Table 1.1. Types of adverse reactions to herbal remedies.

Type	Characteristic	Example
A	Pharmacologically predictable, usually dose dependent	Tachycardia after administration of ephedra
B	Idiosyncratic, not pharmacologically predictable, not dose dependent	Hypersensitivity to a range of herbal medicines
C	Pharmacologically predictable, develop gradually during long-term use	Slowed bowel function after prolonged use of some herbal laxatives
D	Effects with a latency period of months or years	Mutagenic effects of the *Aristolochia* species

the spectrum is too wide for a comprehensive review, examples will be supplied for each of these categories.

1.2 Toxicity of Herbal Ingredients

In principle, herbal medicines have the potential to elicit the same types of adverse reactions as synthetic drugs (Table 1). Consisting of whole extracts of plant parts (e.g. root, leaves), TCHMs contain numerous potentially active molecules. Synergy is often assumed to play a part in the medicinal effects of single plant extracts. Similarly, it is also claimed that combinations of herbs frequently used for TCHM have synergistic effects. There is some *in vitro* and/or *in vivo* evidence to support the occurrence of synergism between constituents in certain herbal extracts; however, direct clinical evidence is largely lacking. The claim of synergy also includes the attenuation of undesirable effects, i.e. the toxicity of plant extracts is less than that of a single isolated constituent. Theoretically, different plant constituents could also interact with each other to render a herbal preparation more toxic than a single chemical constituent. Virtually no evidence is available to substantiate either hypothesis.

The toxicity of herbal ingredients used in TCHM has been more fully reviewed elsewhere (Ernst, 2000b). For the purpose of this article, a few examples in alphabetical order may suffice.

1.3 Aconitum Species (Aconite)

Aconite roots can produce heart failure due to the presence of cardiotoxic alkaloids, such as aconitine. Other symptoms of aconite poisoning are numbing of mouth and tongue, gastrointestinal problems, muscular weakness, lack of coordination and vertigo (Kelly, 1990). A review from Hong Kong reported 17 cases of aconite poisoning after the administration of TCHMs. The toxicity of raw aconite can be decreased substantially by decoction, a process leading to a change in alkaloid composition (Hikino, 1977).

1.4 Aristolochia Species

Plants belonging to the genus of *Aristolochia* are rich in aristolochic acids and aristolactams. Aristolochic acids I and II have mutagenic properties. Aristolactams I and II also show mutagenic activity in bacteria. Aristolochic acids have been demonstrated to pass into human breast milk. High doses of aristolochic acids result in renal toxicity, sometimes even in fatal nephrosis.

In Belgium, an outbreak of nephropathy in about 70 individuals has been attributed to a slimming preparation that supposedly included the Chinese herbs *Stephania tetrandra* and *Magnolia officinalis*. The root of *Stephania tetrandra* (Chinese name "Fangji") was in all probability substituted or contaminated with the root of *Aristolochia fangchi* (Chinese name "Guang fangji") (Vanherweghem *et al.*, 1993; Vanhaelen *et al.*, 1994). The resulting nephropathy was characterised by extensive interstitial fibrosis with atrophy and loss of the tubules (Depierreux *et al.*, 1994) and is today often termed "Chinese herb nephropathy".

In Japan, two cases of Chinese herb nephropathy were associated with chronic use of *Aristolochia manchuriensis* (Kan-modutsu) (Tanaka *et al.*, 2000). The diagnosis was confirmed by renal biopsy and the toxic constituents were identified as aristolochic acids I, II and D. Taiwanese authors have reported 12 cases of suspected Chinese herb nephropathy, confirmed by renal biopsy (Yang *et al.*, 2000). Renal function deteriorated rapidly in most patients, despite withdrawal of the toxic herb. Seven patients underwent dialysis and the rest had slowly progressive renal insufficiency. One patient was subsequently found to have a bladder carcinoma.

Because of fear of malignancies, the Belgian researchers who first described the condition have advocated prophylactic removal of the kidneys and ureters in patients with Chinese herb nephropathy. Of 39 patients who agreed to this, 18 (46%) had urothelial carcinoma, 19 of the others had mild to moderate urothelial dysplasia, and only two had normal urothelium (Nortier *et al.*, 2000). All tissue samples contained aristolochic acid-related DNA in adducts. The original dose of *Aristolochia* correlated positively with the risk of urothelial carcinoma.

More recently, further reports from several countries have confirmed that plants from the aristolochia species cause nephritis (Dai *et al.*, 2001; Tamaki and Okuda, 2001), and the toxic agent was confirmed to be aristolochic acid (Lebeau *et al.*, 2001; Martinez *et al.*, 2002).

A 46-year-old Chinese woman living in Belgium and China was admitted for subacute renal failure (Gillerot, 2001). Her creatine levels had increased from 0.9 mg/dl (November 1998) to 3.7 mg/dl (January 2000). During the preceding six months, she had taken a Chinese patent medicine bought in China "for waste discharging and youth keeping" purposes. The package insert did not disclose any herbs of the aristolochia species. Kidney biopsy showed extensive hypocellular interstitial fibrosis with tubular atrophy and glomerular sclerosis. Analyses of the Chinese medicine demonstrated the presence of aristolochic acid. The patient required haemodialysis in June 2000 and received a renal transplant four months later.

A 58-year-old Japanese woman with calcinosis Raynaud oesophageal sclerodactyly telangiectasia syndrome presented with progressive renal dysfunction (Nishimagi *et al.*, 2001). Renal biopsy showed changes typical for Chinese herb nephropathy. Analyses of the Chinese herbs she had taken for several years demonstrated the presence of aristolochic acid. Therapy with oral prednisolone improved her renal function and anaemia.

1.5 Ephedra Species (Ma Huang)

These contain the tertiary alkaloid ephedrine-producing central and peripheral adrenergic effects such as stimulation, insomnia and tachycardia.

Interference with conventional anti-hypertensive therapy is conceivable. *Ephedra* is used to treat asthma, nasal congestion, fever, obesity and anhidrosis. It is also abused as a recreational drug.

The United States Food and Drug Administration (FDA) database contained 927 cases of adverse effects associated with Ma Huang between 1995 and 1997 (Samenuk *et al.*, 2002). In 16 cases, this was related to stroke, in ten cases to myocardial infarction and in 11 cases to death. Of 140 reports of adverse events related to *Ephedra* supplements submitted to the FDA between June 1997 and March 1999, 31% were definitely or probably caused by *Ephedra* (Haller, 2000). In 47% of the cases, there were cardiovascular symptoms and in 18% central nervous system effects; ten patients died.

1.6 *Ginkgo biloba* (Maidenhair Tree)

Ginkgo is one of the most popular herbal remedies in the West but its origins are, of course, in traditional Chinese medicine. Generally speaking, ginkgo has an excellent safety record which, however, is not to say that it is completely free of adverse effects. A 78-year-old man and an 84-year-old woman with previously well controlled epilepsy presented with recurrent seizures (Granger, 2001). No obvious reason for these events were found and the investigators suspected the self-medication of *Ginkgo biloba* extracts to be the cause. Both patients had started taking ginkgo within two weeks of the onset of the seizures. The herbal remedy was discontinued and both patients remained seizure-free at follow-up several months later. No other change of medication was made. The author postulated that 4-0-methylpyridoxinc, a constituent of ginkgo and a known neurotoxin, was the cause of the seizures.

A 56-year-old man without risk factors suffered a stroke due to a right parietal haematoma (Benjamin *et al.*, 2001). The patient had not taken any medication except for a ginkgo extract (3 × 40 mg/day) which he had started 18 months earlier. On transfer to neurorehabilitation, he still had severe neurological deficits. The authors argue that the antiplatelet effects of ginkgo might have contributed to this case of intracerebral bleeding. A similar case concerns a 78-year-old man who developed a large subdural haematoma after a fall (Miller *et al.*, 2002). The authors believed that ginkgo either caused or predisposed this patient to that complication.

A 34-year-old woman had a laparoscopic cholecystectomy and post-operatively started bleeding into the surgical wound (Fessenden *et al.*, 2001). This led to a fall of haemoglobin from 16.5 to 12.4 g/dl. The patient was given blood transfusions whereupon she recovered uneventfully. The surgeons believe that the woman's self-medication with ginkgo was the cause of this post-operative bleeding. A similar case has been reported where a 59-year-old man developed bleeding complications after a liver transplant (Hauser *et al.*, 2002). The most likely cause was identified to have been the patient's self-medication with a ginkgo supplement.

A 40-year-old African-American female was admitted to the hospital with an exfoliative rash and blistering and swelling of the tongue (Davydov and Stirling, 2001). A diagnosis of Stevens-Johnson Syndrome was made. She had not taken any medication other than two doses of a gingko-containing preparation. Her condition responded to treatment with prednisolone, clotrimazole and famotidine. Ginkgo was discontinued and no further events occurred.

1.7 Ginseng

Ginseng is an ambiguous vernacular term, which may refer to *Panax* species such as *P. ginseng* (Asian ginseng) and *P. quinquefolius* (American ginseng), *Eleutherococcus senticosus* (Siberian ginseng), *Pfaffia paniculata* (Brazilian ginseng) or unidentified material (e.g. Rumanian ginseng). Only the *Panax* species contain ginsenosides. Adverse effects, which have been attributed to ginseng preparations, include hypertension, pressure headaches, dizziness, estrogen-like effects, vaginal bleeding and mastalgia (Thompson Coon and Ernst, 2002). Prolonged use has been associated with a "ginseng abuse syndrome" including symptoms like hypertension, oedema, morning diarrhea, skin eruptions, insomnia, depression and amenorrhea. Inappropriate use has been associated with insomnia, headache, diarrhea as well as cardiovascular and endocrine disorders (Xie *et al.*, 2002). Most reports are difficult to interpret, however, because of the simultaneous use of other agents, insufficient information about dosage and the lack of botanical authentication. The botanical quality of ginseng preparations can be a problem (Cui *et al.*, 1994). For instance, when a case of neonatal androgenisation was associated with maternal use of Siberian ginseng tablets during pregnancy, botanical analysis showed that the incriminated material almost certainly came from *Periploca sepium* (Chinese silk vine) (Awang, 1991). A woman with prior episodes of depression had a manic episode several days after staring to take *Panax ginseng* (Gonzalez-Seijo *et al.*, 1995). Stevens-Johnson syndrome occurred in a 27-year-old man who was a regular user of *Panax ginseng* (Dega *et al.*, 1996). Ginseng has also been associated with a case of cerebral arteritis (Ryu and Chien, 1995).

A 74-year-old man had increased serum digoxin concentrations (without signs of toxicity) while taking Siberian ginseng (McRae, 1996). Common causes of increased serum digoxin were ruled out, and the association with ginseng use was confirmed by de-challenge and re-challenge. The patient's rise in serum digoxin concentration could have been due to cardiac glycosides contained in *Periploca sepium*, a common substitute for *E. senticosus* (Awang, 1996). Diuretic resistance has been reported in a patient consuming a formulation containing *Germanium* and ginseng (species unspecified) (Becker *et al.*, 1996). A case has been reported where the concomitant use of *Panax ginseng* and warfarin resulted in loss of anti-coagulant activity in the latter (Janetzky and Morreale, 1997) (see below). A 56-year-old man presented with a manic episode during *Panax ginseng* intake (Vázquez, 2002). He had no previous history of mental problems. The authors concluded that *Panax ginseng* caused these symptoms of mania.

1.8 *Glycyrrhiza glabra* (Licorice)

The active ingredients of licorice inhibit the breakdown of mineralocorticoids through the inhibition of 11β-hydroxysteroid dehydrogenase type 2. Prolonged use and/or high doses may therefore produce mineralocorticoid adverse effects and drug interactions. These effects are due to the saponin glycoside glycyrrhizin, which is naturally present in licorice root in the form of calcium and potassium salts of glycyrrhizinic acid. Most individuals can consume 400 mg of glycyrrhizin daily without adverse effects, but some individuals will develop adverse effects following regular daily intake of as little as 100 mg of glycyrrhizin (Stormer, 1993). Adverse effects relate mainly to *mineralocorticoid excess*, with sodium retention, potassium loss and inhibition of the renin-angiotensin-aldosterone system (Olukoga and Donaldson, 2000).

In two cases, prolonged intake of relatively small amounts of licorice resulted in *hypertension*, *encephalopathy* and *pseudohyperaldosteronism* (Russo, 2000). When healthy volunteers ingested licorice corresponding to 75–540 mg glycyrrhetinic acid daily for periods of two to four weeks, an average increase of systolic blood pressure of 3.1–14.4 mmHg was noted (Sigurjonsdottir *et al.*, 2001). The authors concluded that 50 g of licorice consumed daily for two weeks causes a significant rise in blood pressure.

The case of a 67-year-old Chinese man presenting with progressive muscle weakness was recently reported (Lin and Chau, 2002). He was diagnosed to have hypokalaemia (2.3 mmol/L) despite treatment with oral potassium chloride, low plasma renin and aldosterone. The cause was identified as his intake of licorice-containing TCHM. His daily dose was equivalent to 336 mg of glycyrrhizic acid per day.

1.9 *Salvia miltiorrhiza* (Danshen)

In China, the root of *Salvia miltiorrhiza* has been use traditionally for the treatment of coronary and other diseases. A pharmacodynamic and pharmacokinetic study in rats suggests that this traditional agent may enhance the anti-coagulant activity of warfarin, when both drugs are taken together. This animal study was initiated because of observations in Hong Kong that patients on routine warfarin therapy experienced an adverse drug interaction when they self-medicated with Danshen (Lo *et al.*, 1992). A patient taking warfarin and who had taken a decoction of *Salvia miltiorrhiza* presented with a prolonged bleeding time and melena (Tam *et al.*, 1995).

1.10 *Tetrahydropalmatine* (Jin Bu Huan)

$_{L}$-*Tetrahydropalmatine* has been identified as the active constituent in Chinese "Jin Bu Huan Anodyne" tablets available on the Western market. The package insert suggested *Polygala chinensis* as source plant, but in reality this alkaloid comes from a *Stephania* species. Both $_{L}$-*Tetrahydropalmatine* and its racemic $_{DL}$-form are used in Chinese medicine as analgesic and hypnotic agents. Reported adverse effects include vertigo, fatigue, nausea and drowsiness. Recent case reports have documented life-threatening bradycardia and respiratory depression in small children following unintentional overdosing (Horowitz *et al.*, 1993) and acute hepatitis in adult users (Woolf *et al.*, 1994).

1.11 Contamination/Adulteration

TCHMs have repeatedly been associated with heavy metal content (Ernst and Thompson Coon, 2001). Several possibilities exist to explain the presence of heavy metals in TCHMs. First, heavy metals could be included intentionally for medicinal properties. Mercury, for instance, is part of some preparations under the term of *cinnabaris* (mercury sulfide) or *calomelas* (mercury chloride). Such products are used for a variety of indications, e.g. as a tranquiliser, an anti-epileptic agent, for ulcers, or to treat insomnia (Koh and Woo, 2000). Lead is used and termed as *mi tuo seng* (lithargyrum) (Zhu, 1998) and arsenic as *xiong huang* (Realgar) (Chinese Pharmacopoeia Commission of the Ministry of Public Health, 1997) in the manufacture of some TCHMs.

Second, the presence of heavy metals may be the result of accidental contamination during manufacture, for instance, from grinding weights or lead-releasing containers or other manufacturing utensils (Koh and Woo, 2000). Third, medicinal herbs may contain heavy metals when grown in seriously polluted soil (Schilcher, 1983). In this context it is relevant to note that TCHMs may also contain animal and mineral products and that these may also be contaminated with heavy metals (Chuang *et al.*, 2000).

The results of a systematic review (Ernst and Thompson Coon, 2001) show that heavy metal poisoning through TCHM use has been reported with some regularity (Chan and Critchley, 1996; Tay and Seah, 1975; Lightfoote *et al.*, 1997; Chan *et al.*, 2001; Levit *et al.*, 1984; Yu and Yeung, 1987; Schaumburg and Berger, 1992; Kang-yum and Oransky, 1992; Markowitz *et al.*, 1994; Wu, 1996a and b; Wong *et al.*, 1998a and b; Cuncha *et al.*, 1998; Li *et al.*, 2000). Moreover, epidemiologic (Chu, 1998; Cheng *et al.*, 1998) and analytical (Myerson *et al.*, 1982; D'Alauro *et al.*, 1984; Chi *et al.*, 1992; Espinoza, 1995) investigations have shown that a considerable proportion of TCHMs contains heavy metals. Severe clinical consequences (Wu, 1996a and b; Wong *et al.*, 1998a) and even fatalities (Tay and Seah, 1975; Kang-yum and Oransky, 1992; Wong *et al.*, 1998b; Cuncha *et al.*, 1998) are on record. Children are particularly vulnerable and have been involved relatively often (Tay and Seah, 1975; Chan *et al.*, 2001; Levit *et al.*, 1984; Yu and Yeung, 1987; Kang-yum and Oransky, 1992; Cuncha *et al.*, 1998; Li *et al.*, 2000). In many cases, (Tay and Seah, 1975; Lightfoote *et al.*, 1997; Chan *et al.*, 2001; Yu and Yeung, 1987; Schaumburg and Berger, 1992; Kang-yum and Oransky, 1992; Markowitz *et al.*, 1994;

Table 1.2. Synthetic drugs identified in TCHMs.

Aminopyrine
Clobetasolpropionate
Dexametasone
Diazepam
Diclofenac
Fluocinoloneacetonide
Fluocortolone
Glibenclamide
Hydrochlorothiazide
Hydrocortisone
Indomethacin
Menfenamic acid
Methylsalicylate
Phenacetin
Phenylbutazone
Prednisolone

Wu, 1996a and b; Wong *et al.*, 1998a and b) TCHM intake had been prolonged until a diagnosis of intoxication was made. Intoxications have also been documented in the West (Lightfoote *et al.*, 1997; Schaumburg and Berger, 1992; Kang-yum and Oransky, 1992; Markowitz *et al.*, 1994). Other potential contaminants of TCHMs include toxic botanicals (see above), micro-organisms, microbial toxins, pesticides and fumigation agents (De Smet, 2002).

Numerous instances are on record where TCHMs have been adulterated with synthetic drugs. Table 2 lists such ingredients identified in a recent systematic review of the subject (Ernst, 2002a). One fatality (Ries and Sahud, 1975) and several potentially life-threatening events have repeatedly been documented (Forster *et al.*, 1979; Offerhaus and Dukes, 1979; Hughes *et al.*, 1994; Stricht *et al.*, 1994; Goudie and Kaye, 2001).

1.12 TCHM-Drug Interactions

Interaction can be either pharmacodynamic or pharmacokinetic by nature. In the former case, both interacting medicines typically have the same pharmacological effects; the result would be an exaggerated clinical response. In the latter case, one medicine interferes with the absorption, distribution, metabolism or excretion of the other; the result would be an exaggeration or diminution of the clinical response.

A recent systematic review (Fugh-Berman and Ernst, 2001) of all documented cases of herb-drug interactions comprised 11 instances of clinical events (Tam, 1995; Izzat, 1998; Yu, 1997; Page, 1999; Ellis, 1999; Galluzi *et al.*, 2000; Matthews, 1998; Rosenblatt and Mindel, 1997; Janetzky and Morreale, 1997; Jones, 1987; Shader, 1985). Their details are summarised in Table 3. Virtually all interactions concern the blood coagulation system. The reason might be that anti-coagulated patients are closely monitored. Thus interactions might affect other physiological functions but remain unnoticed. In addition to these documented clinical cases, numerous herbal medicines have the potential of interacting with synthetic drugs (Ernst, 2000a).

Table 1.3. Case reports of interactions between TCHMs and synthetic drugs.

Patient description (Reference)	Herb Latin name	Synthetic drug	Concomitant medications	Signs or symptoms of interaction	Mechanism	Causality
66-year-old man with atrial fibrillation, rheumatic mitral stenosis, cerebral embolism and gastric adenocarcinoma (Tam, 1995)	Danshen *Salvia miltiorrhiza*	Warfarin	Digoxin, propranolol, topical oil containing 15% salicylates	↑ INR; gastric bleeding	Probably no interaction but additive action due to coumarin content of herb	Possible
62-year-old man with mitral valve replacement (Izzat, 1998)	Danshen *Salvia miltiorrhiza*	Warfarin	Digoxin, furosemide, captopril	↑ INR	Probably no interaction but additive action due to coumarin content of herb	Likely
48-year-old woman with a history of rheumatic heart disease, mitral stenosis and atrial fibrillation (Yu, 1997)	Danshen *Salvia miltiorrhiza*	Warfarin	Digoxin, furosemide, theophylline, mefenamic acid	↑ INR	Probably no interaction but additive action due to coumarin content of herb	Possible

Table 1.3. (*Continued*)

Patient description (Reference)	Herb Latin name	Synthetic drug	Concomitant medications	Signs or symptoms of interaction	Mechanism	Causality
46-year-old woman with history of stroke, rheumatic heart disease and atrial fibrillation (Page, 1999)	Dong quai *Angelica sinensis*	Warfarin	Digoxin, furosemide	$\uparrow$ INR	Herb acts as Cox inhibitor	Likely
Woman with history of mitral valve replacement (Ellis, 1999)	Dong quai *Angelica sinensis*	Warfarin	None stated	INR = 10, widespread bruising	Herb acts as Cox inhibitor	Possible
80-year-old Alzheimer's patient (Galluzi *et al.*, 2000)	Ginkgo *Ginkgo biloba*	Trazodone	Bromazepam, donepezil, vitamin E discontinued within 3 days	Coma	Herb has anti-platelet activity	Possible
78-year-old woman with history of hypertension, myocardial infarction, atrial fibrillation, coronary bypass and gait problems (Matthews, 1998)	Ginkgo *Ginkgo biloba*	Warfarin	None stated	PT 16.9, PTT 35.5, left parietal haemorrhage	Herb has anti-platelet activity	Possible

(*Continued*)

Table 1.3. Case reports of interactions between TCHMs and synthetic drugs (*Continued*).

Patient description (Reference)	Herb Latin name	Synthetic drug	Concomitant medications	Signs or symptoms of interaction	Mechanism	Causality
70-year-old man with history of coronary artery bypass (no other details) (Rosenblatt and Mindel, 1997)	Ginkgo *Ginkgo biloba*	Aspirin	None stated	Spontaneous hyphema (bleeding into the iris)	Herb has anti-platelet activity	Possible
47-year-old man with history of heart valve replacement (Janetzky and Morreale, 1997)	Ginseng *Panax* species	Warfarin	Diltiazem, nitroglycerine, salsalate	INR decreased to 1.5 (previously stable 2–3)	Herb has anti-platelet activity	Likely
42-year-old woman with chronic depression (Jones, 1987)	Ginseng *Panax* species	Phenelzine	Lorazepam, triazolam, bee pollen	Manic symptoms	n.k.	Possible
64-year-old woman (Shader, 1985)	Ginseng *Panax* species	Phenelzine	None	Insomnia, headache, tremor	n.k.	Unevaluable

INR = International Normalised Ratio.
n.k. = Not known.

1.13 Discussion

The evidence cited above shows that TCHM is not risk-free. This begs the question as to the size of the problem. Unfortunately reliable incidence figures of adverse events are presently not available.

A study of 1701 patients admitted to two general wards of a Hong Kong hospital revealed that three (0.2%) of these cases were due to adverse reactions to TCHMs; two of the three cases were serious (Chan *et al.*, 1992). A retrospective study of all 2695 patients admitted to a Taiwanese department of medicine during a period of ten months showed that 4% of these patients were admitted because of drug-related problems, and that TCHM ranked third amongst the categories of medicines responsible (Lin and Lin, 1993). An active surveillance adverse drug reaction reporting programme conducted in a family medicine ward of the National Taiwan University Hospital reported that TCHMs were responsible for five (22% of total) hospital admissions or 12% of all adverse drug reactions observed in the study (Wu *et al.*, 1996).

When 1100 Australian practitioners of traditional Chinese medicine were asked to complete questionnaires about the adverse effects of TCHMs, they reported 860 adverse events, including 19 deaths (Bensoussan *et al.*, 2000). It was calculated that each practitioner had encountered an average of 1.4 adverse events during each year of full-time practice.

A physician prospectively monitored all 1265 patients taking TCHMs at his clinic during 33 months (Al-Khafaji, 2000). Liver enzymes were measured before the start of therapy and three and ten weeks later. Alanin aminotransferase activity was raised in 107 patients (8.5%) who initially had normal values. Of these patients, about 25% reported symptoms such as abdominal discomfort, looseness of bowels, loss of appetite, or fatigue.

These data show that the frequency of adverse effects is variable. As denominator data are largely missing, incidence figures are not definable. Good quality studies on the toxicity of TCHM are also lacking, both in the Chinese as well as the non-Chinese literature (Bensoussan *et al.*, 2002). Thus the creation of a systematic toxicology database of TCHMs is a laudable and important step towards increasing consumers' safety. To date, 12 monographs are available in this database.

The evidence cited above relies mostly on case reports. Thus it is intrinsically weak and causality is often uncertain. It follows that more systematic research would be highly desirable. Until it becomes available it might be wise to be cautious particularly when using TCHMs for vulnerable individuals such as the elderly (Ernst, 2002b), pregnant/lactating women (Ernst, 2002c) and children (Ernst, 2003). Clinicians "must tread a line between an apparently sympathetic stance that might be interpreted as an endorsement of unproven therapies and categorical disapproval, which would discourage patients from revealing their use of herbal remedies" (De Smet, 2002).

In conclusion, TCHMs are not devoid of risk. In the interest of consumer safety, the systematic study of this subject should be encouraged.

References

Al-Khafaji, M. (2000) Monitoring of liver enzymes in patients on Chinese medicine. *J. Chin. Med.* **62**, 6–10.

Awang, D.V.C. (1991) Maternal use of ginseng and neonatal androgenisation. *JAMA* **155**, 266.

Awang, D.V.C. (1996) Siberian ginseng toxicity may be case of mistaken identity. *Can. Med. Assoc. J.* **155**, 1237.

Becker, B.N., Greene, J., Evanson, J., Chidsey, G. and Stone, W.J. (1996) Ginseng-induced diuretic resistance. *JAMA* **276**, 606–607.

Benjamin, J., Muir, T., Briggs, K. and Pentland, B. (2001) A case of cerebral haemorrhage — can *Ginkgo biloba* be implicated? *Postgrad. Med. J.* **77**, 112–113.

Bensoussan, A, Myers, S.P. and Carlton, A.-L. (2000) Risks associated with the practice of traditional Chinese medicine. *Arch. Fam. Med.* **9**, 1071–1078.

Bensoussan, A., Myers, S.P., Drew, A.K., Whyte, I.M. and Dawson, A.H. (2002) Development of a Chinese herbal medicine toxicology database. *Clin. Toxicol.* **40**, 159–167.

Chan, H., Yen, Y.-Y., Billmeier, G.J. and Evans, W.E. (2001) Lead poisoning from ingestion of Chinese herbal medicine. *Clin. Toxicol.* **10**, 273–281.

Chan, T.Y.K. and Critchley, J.A. (1996) Usage and adverse effects of Chinese herbal medicines. *Hum. Exp. Toxicol.* **15**, 5–12.

Chan, T.Y.K., Chan, A.Y. and Critchley, J.A. (1992) Hospital admissions due to adverse reactions to Chinese herbal medicines. *J. Trop. Med. Hyg.* **95**, 296–298.

Cheng, T., Wong, R., Lin, Y., Hwang, Y., Horng, J. and Wang, J. (1998) Chinese herbal medicine, sibship, and blood lead in children. *Occup. Environ. Med.* **55**, 573–576.

Chi, Y.W., Chen, S.L., Yang, M.H., Hwang, R.C. and Chu, M.L. (1992) Survey of heavy metals in traditional Chinese medicinal preparations. *Chin. Med. J.* **50**, 400–405.

Chu, J.F. (1998) Risk factors for high blood lead levels among the general population in Taiwan. *Eur. J. Epidemiol.* **14**, 775–781.

Chuang, I.C., Chen, K.-S., Huang, Y.-L., Lee, P.-N. and Lin, T.-H. (2000) Determination of trace elements in some natural drugs by atomic absorption spectrometry. *Biol. Trace Elem. Res.* **76**, 235–244.

Cui, J., Garle, M., Eneroth, P. and Björkhem, I. (1994) What do commercial ginseng preparations contain? *Lancet* **344**, 134.

Cuncha, J., Pereira, L., Pun, M.I., Lopes, V. and Vong, S.K. (1998) Arsenic and acute lethal intoxication. *Hong Kong Pharm. J.* **7**, 50–53.

D'Alauro, F., Lin-Fu, J.S. and Ecker, T.J. (1984) Toxic metal contamination of folk remedy. *JAMA* **252**, 3127.

Dai, X.-W., Rao, X.-R. and Li, S. (2001) Current situation of Chinese herb-induced renal damage and its countermeasures. *CJIM* **7**, 162–166.

Davydov, L. and Stirling, A.L. (2001) Stevens-Johnson syndrome with *Ginkgo biloba*. *J. Herb. Pharmacother.* **1**, 65–69.

De Smet, P.A.G.M. (2002) Herbal remedies. *N. Engl. J. Med.* **347**, 2046–2056.

Dega, H., Laporte, J.-L., Francès, C., Herson, S. and Chosidow, O. (1996) Ginseng as a cause for Stevens-Johnson syndrome. *Lancet* **347**, 1344.

Depierreux, M., Van Damme, B., Vanden Houte, K. and Vanherweghem, J.L. (1994) Pathologic aspects of a newly described nephropathy related to the prolonged used of Chinese herbs. *Am. J. Kidney Dis.* **24**, 172–180.

Ellis, G.R. (1999) Untitled (photograph and brief case report). In "Minerva". *Br. Med. J.* **319**, 650.

Ernst, E. (2000a) Interactions between synthetic and herbal medicinal products. Part 2: a systematic review of the indirect evidence. *Perfusion* **13**, 60–70.

Ernst, E. (2000b) Risks associated with complementary therapies. In: *Meyler's Side Effects of Drugs*, 14th Ed. (eds.) Dukes, M.N.G. and Aronson, J.K. Elsevler, Amsterdam, pp. 1649–1681.

Ernst, E. (2002a) Adulteration of Chinese herbal medicines with synthetic drugs: a systematic review. *J. Intern. Med.* **251**, 107–113.

Ernst, E. (2002b) Adverse effects of unconventional therapies in the elderly: a systematic review of the recent literature. *J. Am. Aging Assoc.* **25**, 11–20.

Ernst, E. (2002c) Herbal medicinal products during pregnancy: are they safe? *Int. J. Obstet. Gynecol.* **109**, 227–235.

Ernst, E. (2003) Serious adverse effects of unconventional therapies for children and adolescents: a systematic review of recent evidence. *Eur. J. Pediatr.* **162**, 72–80.

Ernst, E. and Thompson Coon, J. (2001) Heavy metals in traditional Chinese medicines: a systematic review. *Clin. Pharmacol. Ther.* **70**, 497–504.

Espinoza, E.O. (1995) Arsenic and mercury in traditional Chinese herbal balls. *N. Engl. J. Med.* **333**, 803–804.

Fessenden, M., Wittenborn, W. and Clarke, L. (2001) *Ginkgo biloba*: a case report of herbal medicine and bleeding postoperatively from a laparoscopic cholecystectomy. *Am. Surg.* **67**, 33–35.

Forster, P.G.J., Calverley, M., Hubball, S. and McConkey, B. (1979) Chuei-Fong-Tou-Geu-Wan in rheumatoid arthritis. *Br. Med. J.* **ii**, 308.

Fugh-Berman, A. and Ernst, E. (2001) Herb-drub interactions: review and assessment of report reliability. *Br. J. Clin. Pharmacol.* **52**, 587–595.

Galluzi, S., Zanetti, O., Binetti, G., *et al.* (2000) Coma in a patient with Alzheimer's disease taking low dose trazodone and *Ginkgo biloba*. *J. Neurol. Neurosurg. Psych.* **68**, 679–683.

Gillerot, G., Jadoul, M., Arlt, V.M., Van, Y., De Strihou, C., Schmeiser, H.M., But, P.P.H., *et al.* (2001) Aristolochic acid nephropathy in a Chinese patient: time to abandon the term "Chinese herbs nephropathy"? *Am. J. Kidney Dis.* **38**, 1–5.

Gonzalez-Seijo, J.C., Kamos, Y.M. and Lastra, I. (1995) Manic episode and ginseng: report of a possible case. *J. Clin. Psychopharmacol.* **15**, 447–478.

Goudie, A.M. and Kaye, J.M. (2001) Contaminated medication precipitating hypoglycaemia. *Med. J. Aust.* **175**, 257.

Granger, A.S. (2001) *Ginkgo biloba* precipitating epileptic seizures. *Age Ageing* **30**, 523–525.

Haller, C.A. (2000) Adverse cardiovascular and central nervous system events associated with dietary supplements containing ephedra alkaloids. *N. Engl. J. Med.* **343**, 1833–1838.

Hauser, D., Gayowski, T. and Singh, H. (2002) Bleeding complications precipitated by unrecognised *Gingko biloba* use after liver transplantation. *Transpl. Int.* **15**, 377–379.

Hikino, H., Yamada, C. and Nakamura, K. (1977) Change of alkaloid composition and acute toxicity of *Aconitum* roots during processing. *Yakugaku Zasshi* **97**, 359.

Horowitz, R.S., Gomez, H., Moore, L.L., Fulton, B., Feldhaus, K., Brent, J., *et al.* (1993) Jin Bu Huan toxicity in children — Colorado. *Morb. Mortal. Weekly Rep.* **42**, 633–636.

Hughes, J.R., Higgins, E.M. and Pembroke, A.C. (1994) Oral dexamethasone masquerading as a Chinese herbal remedy. *Br. J. Dermatol.* **130**, 261.

Izzat, M.B. (1998) A taste of Chinese medicine. *Ann. Thorac. Surg.* **66**, 941.

Janetzky, K. and Morreale, A.P. (1997) Probable interactions between warfarin and ginseng. *Am. J. Health Syst. Pharm.* **54**, 692–693.

Jones, B.D. (1987) Interaction of ginseng with phenelzine. *J. Clin. Psychopharmacol.* **7**, 201–202.

Kang-yum, E. and Oransky, S.H. (1992) Chinese patent medicine as a potential source of mercury poisoning. *Vet. Hum. Toxicol.* **34**, 235–238.

Kelly, S.P. (1990) Aconite poisoning. *Med. J. Aust.* **153**, 499.

Koh, H.-L. and Woo, S.-O. (2000) Chinese proprietary medicine in Singapore. Regulatory control of toxic heavy metals and undeclared drugs. *Drug Saf.* **23**, 351–362.

Lebeau, C., Arlt, V.M., Schmeiser, H.H., Boom, A., Verroust, P.J., Devuyst, O., *et al.* (2001) Aristolochic acid impedes endocytosis and induces DNA adducts in proximal tubule cells. *Kidney Int.* **60**, 1332–1342.

Levit, C., Godes, J., Ing, R. and Simpson, J.M. (1984) Sources of lead poisoning. *JAMA* **252**, 3127–3128.

Li, A.M., Chan, M.H.M., Leung, T.F., Cheung, R.C.K., Lam, C.W.K. and Fok, T.F. (2000) Mercury intoxication presenting with tics. *Arch. Dis. Child.* **83**, 174–175.

Lightfoote, J., Blaire, J. and Cohen, J.R. (1997) Lead intoxication in an adult caused by Chinese herbal medication. *JAMA* **238**, 1539.

Lin, C.H., Chang, S.H. and Hsu, H.C. (2000) Rapidly progressing fibrosing interstitial nephritis associated with Chinese herbal drugs. *Am. J. Kidney Dis.* **35**, 313–318.

Lin, S. and Chau, T. (2002) A puzzling cause of hypokalaemia. *Lancet* **360**, 224.

Lin, S.H. and Lin, M.S. (1993) A survey on drug related hospitalisation in a community teaching hospital. *Int. J. Clin. Pharmacol. Ther. Toxicol.* **31**, 66–69.

Lo, A.C.T., Chan, K.M., Yeung, J.H.K. and Woo, K.S. (1992) The effects of Danshen (*Salvia miltiorrhiza*) on pharmacokinetics and pharmacodynamics of warfarin in rats. *Eur. J. Drug Metab. Pharmacokin.* **17**, 257–262.

Markowitz, S.B., Nunez, C.M., Klitzman, S., Munski, A.A., Kim, W.S., Eisinger, J., *et al.* (1994) Lead poisoning due to Hai Ge Fen. *JAMA* **271**, 932–934.

Martinez, M., Nortier, J., Vereerstraeten, P. and Vanherweghem, J. (2002) Progression rate of Chinese herb nephropathy: impact of *Aristolochia fangchi* ingested dose. *Nephrol. Dial. Transplant.* **17**, 408–412.

Matthews, M.K. (1998) Association of *Ginkgo biloba* with intracerebral haemorrhage. *Neurology* **5**, 1933.

McRae, S. (1996) Elevated serum digoxin levels in a patient taking digoxin and Siberian ginseng. *Can. Med. Ass. J.* **155**, 293–295.

Miller, L.G. and Freeman, B. (2002) Subdural hematoma associated with *Ginkgo biloba*. *J. Herb. Pharmacother.* **2**, 57–63.

Myerson, G.E., Myerson, A.S., Miller, S.B., Goldman, J.A. and Wilson, C.H. (1982) Chinese herbal medicine mail order syndrome [abstract]. *Arthritis Rheum.* **25**, S87–S87.

Nishimagi, E., Kawaguchi, Y., Terai, C., Kajiyama, H., Hara, M. and Kamatani, N. (2001) Progressive interstitial renal fibrosis due to Chinese herbs in a patient with calcinosis Raynaud esophageal sclerodactyly telangiectasia (CREST) syndrome. *Intern. Med.* **40**, 1059–1063.

Nortier, J.L. and Martinez, M. (2000) Urothelial carcinoma associated with the use of a Chinese herb (*Aristolochia fangchi*). *N. Engl. J. Med.* **342**, 1686–1692.

Offerhaus, L. and Dukes, M.N.G. (1979) "Herbal" medicines and rheumatoid arthritis. *Br. Med. J.* **ii**, 668.

Olukoga, A. and Donaldson, D. (2000) Liquorice and its health implications. *J. Roy. Soc. Promot. Health* **120**, 83–89.

Page, R.L. (1999) Potentiation of warfarin by Dong Quai. *Pharmacotherapy* **19**, 870–876.

Ries, C.A. and Sahud, M.A. (1975) Agranulocytosis caused by Chinese herbal medicines. *JAMA* **231**, 352–355.

Rosenblatt, M. and Mindel, J. (1997) Spontaneous hyphema associated with ingestion of *Ginkgo biloba* extract. *N. Engl. J. Med.* **April 10**, 1108.

Russo, S. (2000) Low dose of liquorice can induce hypertension encephalopathy. *Am. J. Nephrol.* **20**, 145–148.

Ryu, S.-J. and Chien, Y.-Y. (1995) Ginseng-associated cerebral arteritis. *Neurology* **45**, 829–830.

Samenuk, D., Link, M.S., Homoud, M.K., Contreras, R., Theohardes, T.C., Wang, P.J., *et al.* (2002). Adverse cardiovascular events temporally associated with Ma Huang, an herbal source of ephedrine. *Mayo Clin. Proc.* **77**, 12–16.

Schaumburg, H.H. and Berger, A. (1992) Alopecia and sensory polyneuropathy from thallium in a Chinese herbal medication. *JAMA* **268**, 3430–3431.

Scheid, V. (2000) The globalisation of Chinese medicine. *Lancet* **354**, 10.

Schilcher, H. (1983) Contamination of natural products with pesticides and heavy metals. In: *Topics in Pharmaceutical Sciences*, (eds.) Breimer, D.D. and Speiser, P. Elsevier Science, Amsterdam, pp. 417–423.

Shader, R.I. (1985) Phenelzine and the dream machine — ramblings and reflections. *J. Clin. Psychopharmacol.* **5**, 65.

Sigurjonsdottir, H.A., Franzson, L., Manhem, K., Ragnarsson, J., Sigurdsson, G. and Wallerstedt, S. (2001) Liquorice-induced rise in blood pressure: a linear dose-response relationship. *J. Hum. Hypertens.* **15**, 549–552.

Stormer, F.C. (1993) Glycyrrhizic acid in liquorice — evaluation of health hazard. *Food Chem. Toxicol.* **31**, 303–312.

Stricht, B.V., Parvais, O.E., Vanhaelen-Fastré, R.J. and Vanhaelen, M.H. (1994) Remedies may contain cocktail of active drugs. *Br. Med. J.* **308**, 1162.

Tam, L.S. (1995) Warfarin interactions with Chinese traditional medicines: danshen and methyl-salicylate medicated oil. *Aust. NZ J. Med.* **25**, 258.

Tam, L.S., Chan, T.Y.K., Leung, W.K. and Critchley, J.A. (1995) Warfarin interactions with Chinese traditional medicines: danshen and methyl salicylate medicated oil. *Aust. NZ J. Med.* **25**, 258.

Tamaki, K. and Okuda, S. (2001) Chinese herbs nephropathy: a variant form in *Japan. Intern. Med.* **40**, 267–268.

Tanaka, A., Nishida, R., Maeda, K., Sugawara, A. and Kuwahara, T. (2000) Chinese herb nephropathy in Japan presents adult-onset Fanconi syndrome: could different components of aristolochic acids cause a different type of Chinese herb nephropathy? *Clin. Nephrol.* **53**, 301–306.

Tay, C.H. and Seah, C.S. (1975) Arsenic poisoning from anti-asthmatic herbal preparations. *Med. J. Aus.* **2**, 424–428.

The Chinese Pharmacopoeia Commission of the Ministry of Public Health (1997) *Pharmacopoeia of the People's Republic of China*, 1997 Ed., Vol. 1. Guangdong Technology and Chemical Industries, Guangdong.

Thompson Coon, J. and Ernst, E. (2002) *Panax ginseng*: a systematic review of adverse effects and drug interactions. *Drug. Saf.* **25**, 323–344.

Vanhaelen, M., Vanhaelen-Fastre, R., But, P. and Vanherweghem, J.L. (1994) Identification of aristolochic acid in Chinese herbs. *Lancet* **343**, 174.

Vanherweghem, J.L., Depierreux, M., Tielemans, C., Abramowicz, D., Dratwa, M., Jadoul, M., *et al.* (1993) Rapidly progressive interstitial renal fibrosis in young women: association with slimming regimen including Chinese herbs. *Lancet* **341**, 387–391.

Vázquez, A. (2002) Herbal products and serious side effects: a case of ginseng-induced manic episode. *Acta Psychiatr.* **105**, 76–78.

Wong, S.T., Chan, H.L. and Teo, S.K. (1998) The spectrum of cutaneous and internal malignancies in chronic arsenic toxicity. *Singapore Med. J.* **39**, 171–173.

Woolf, G.M., Petrovic, L.M., Rojter, S.E., Wainwright, S., Villamil, F.G., Katkov, W.N., *et al.* (1994) Acute hepatitis associated with the Chinese herbal product Jin Bu Huan. *Ann. Intern. Med.* **121**, 729–735.

Wu, F.-L., Yang, C.-C., Shen, L.-J. and Chen, C.-Y. (1996) Adverse drug reactions in a medical ward. *J. Formos. Med. Assoc.* **95**, 241–246.

Wu, M.S. (1996a) Multiple tubular dysfunction induced by mixed Chinese herbal medicines containing cadmium. *Nephrol. Dial. Transplant.* **11**, 867–870.

Wu, T.N. (1996b) Lead poisoning caused by contaminated Cordyceps, a Chinese herbal medicine: two case reports. *Sci. Total Environ.* **182**, 193–195.

Wong, S.S., Tan, K.C. and Goh, C.L. (1998) Cutaneous manifestations of chronic arsenicism: review of 17 cases. *J. Am. Acad. Dermatol.* **Feb**, 179–185.

Wong, S.T., Chan, H.L. and Teo, S.K. (1998) The spectrum of cutaneous and internal malignancies in chronic arsenic toxicity. *Singapore Med. J.* **39**, 171–173.

Xie, J.-T., Mehendale, S.R., Maleckar, S.A. and Yuan, C.-S. (2002) Is ginseng free from adverse effects? *Orient. Pharm. Exp. Med.* **2**, 80–86.

Yang, C.S., Lin, C.H., Chang, S.H. and Hsu, H.C. (2000) Rapidly progressing fibrosing interstitial nephritis associated with Chinese herbal drugs. *Am. J. Kidney Dis.* **35**, 313–318.

Yu, C.M. (1997) Chinese herbs and warfarin potentiation by Danshen. *J. Intern. Med.* **241**, 337–339.

Yu, E.C.L. and Yeung, C.Y. (1987) Lead encephalopathy due to herbal medicine. *Chinese Med. J.* **100**, 915–917.

Zhu, Y.P. (1998) Chinese Materia Medica: Chemistry, Pharmacology and Applications. Harwood Academic Publishers, Amsterdam.

Chapter 2

Research of Acupuncture Ameliorating Psycho-Craving for Patients Dependent on Heroin

Jun-mei Wu, Jian-hua Lin, Yong-fen Luo & Jun Li

Abstract

The authors examined the results of using acupuncture in de-addiction of opium with buprenorphine and opium with Hans instrument for de-addiction, and studied its mechanism. The results showed the dominance of acu-treatment for controlling craving after 8 days. It suggested the use of acupuncture for treating the psychic dependence during the period between the stages of abstinence and rehabilitation.

Keywords: Acupuncture; Heroin Dependence; Stage of Abstinence; Opium; Buprenorphine; Craving; Hans Instrument for De-addiction; Withdrawal Syndrome.

2.1 Introduction

There is a high relapse rate in heroin de-addiction, usually over 95% within half a year (Zhang, 1997). It is a very big problem in treating heroin dependence. Relapse is mainly caused by withdrawal syndrome and craving. There are two kinds of medicines with different therapeutic mechanism that are used in the stage of recovery: one is methadone, an opioid receptor agonist — this medicine should not be used widely since it may cause dependence itself; the other is naltrexone, an opiate antagonist — this medicine could force addicts to give up heroin transiently by blocking the euphoric effects of exogenously administered opioids, controlling craving, alleviating positive reinforcement of heroin, causing no dependence after detoxification and alleviating negative reinforcement of heroin. But there is a difference between the concept of "give up compulsively" and that of "do not want". And this difference is the reason why a lot of addicts take heroin straight after they are released from prisons. Therefore, many researchers are seeking methods of preventing relapse using Chinese medicine. This study was designed to investigate the addicts' experience when receiving acupuncture as a treatment for heroin dependence in conjunction with other conventional treatment modalities.

2.2 Material

2.2.1 *Subjects*

All subjects were addicts voluntarily or compulsively, who were receiving de-addiction treatment in the Institute of Compulsive De-addiction of Qingyang Branch of Chengdu Public Security Bureau. All subjects met the following conditions: (1) criteria for a diagnosis of opioid dependence in the second edition of *The Classification and Diagnosis Standard of Chinese Psychiatry* (*CCMD-2-R*), which is published by the Psychiatric Association of Chinese Medical Association, and the related diagnosis in the revised third edition of *Diagnostic and Statistical Manual of Mental Disorders* (*DSM-III-R*), which is published by the American Psychiatric Association; (2) still using heroin; and (3) positive results in the urine test of heroin qualitative analysis. The subjects were excluded if they had complications, infectious diseases or psychoses, below 18 years old, over 60 years old or pregnant.

2.2.2 *Main reagents and apparatus*

The reagents and apparatus include: detection reagent for urine screening test for heroin (produced in the US, bought from Beijing Shai Fu Er Ke Mao Company Limited); LH-201 Hans instrument for de-addiction (produced by the Chinese National Medical Appliance Company and Beijing Pu Kang Medical Scientific Development Company); disposable sterile needles (produced by Suzhou Medical Appliance Factory); opium and buprenorphine (produced by Qinghai Pharmaceutical Factory).

2.3 Methods

2.3.1 *Grouping*

The subjects who voluntarily accepted de-addiction treatment were divided into groups of opium with buprenorphine according to the heroin consumed per day: 18 subjects with less than 0.5 g per day; 6 subjects with more than 0.5 g but less than 1.0 g per day; and 6 subjects with equal or more than 1.0 g per day.

The subjects who were compelled to accept treatment, were randomised into another three groups: opium with acupuncture, acupuncture, and opium with Hans instrument. According to the *Guide Principle of De-addiction Methods for Opium Addiction* published by the Ministry of Health, the period of treatment was ten days (from the last time consuming drugs, 24 hours is a day.)

2.3.2 *Treatment*

The groups of opium with buprenorphine were given a fixed formula used in the Institute of Compulsive De-addiction of Qingyang Branch of Chengdu Public Security Bureau, which consists of tapering doses of opium (100 mg per time, three times per day for the first three days, 50 mg per time and three times per day from the fourth day to the sixth day, 50 mg per time and twice per day from the seventh day to ninth day, and only 50 mg before sleep on the tenth day). Moreover, a drip was set with buprenorphine 0.3 mg into 5% Dextrose 500 ml and buprenorphine intramuscular injection 0.15 mg before sleep on the first two days, buprenorphine intramuscular injection 0.15 mg every 12 hours on the third day, buprenorphine intramuscular injection 0.15 mg before sleep on the fourth day. Chlorpromazine of 100 mg is required to be orally taken before sleep every day.

The groups of acupuncture were given a formula that includes Sishencong, Neiguan (PC 6), Hegu (LI 4), Zusanli (ST 36), Sanyinjiao

(SP 6). Additional points are chosen according to differential diagnosis. Renzhong or manipulation of puncturing Zhiyang (GV 9) and cupping were used when necessary. All acupuncture manipulation was performed by the authors. Even reinforcing and reducing movement was used on Sishencong; reducing movement by lifting and thrusting the needle was manipulated and repeated three times on Neiguan and Hegu; the method of "setting the mountain on fire" was used on Zusanli; reinforcing movement by lifting and thrusting the needle was manipulated and repeated three times on Sanyinjiao. All needles were retained for 30 minutes with stimulation of the acupuncture point every five minutes after "Deqi" sensation was elicited. The treatment was performed twice per day on the first three days (first time at 9–11 o'clock in the morning, the other at 3–5 o'clock in the afternoon, and once more at 9–11 o'clock at night when necessary) and once a day during the last 7 days (at 3–5 o'clock in the afternoon). The placebo was made by amylum with the same colour, size and taking method as opium and chlorpromazine.

In the groups of opium with acupuncture, the method of administering a tapering dose of opium was the same as the method used in the group of opium with buprenorphine. The treatment of acupuncture was similar to the group of acupuncture. Chlorpromazine was taken before sleep at a dosage of 100 mg every day.

In the group of opium with Hans instrument, the method of administering a tapering dose of opium was the same as used in the group of opium with buprenorphine. Acupoints used for Hans instrument were Hegu (LI 4), Laogong (PC 8), Zusanli (ST 36) and Sanyinjiao (SP 6). Treatment was administered thrice during the first three days (4- to 6-hour interval) and twice during the last 7 days (8-hour interval). Chlorpromazine was taken before sleep at a dosage of 100 mg every day.

2.3.3 *Observation method*

The visual analog scale (VAS) was used to measure the craving feelings (Ge *et al.*, 1995). Participants rated their craving feelings on the VAS from "no craving feelings at all" (0 mm) to "severe craving" (100 mm) every day from the last time taking heroin.

Table 2.1. Visual Analogue Scale Craving Feelings (%).

Treatment time (day)	Group of opium with buprenorphine	Group of acupuncture	Group of opium with acupuncture	Group of opium with Hans instrument
	N = 30	N = 30	N = 30	N = 30
1	47.40 ± 35.62	58.43 ± 34.86	63.15 ± 31.35	62.98 ± 33.96
2	42.91 ± 33.21	50.25 ± 35.84	46.27 ± 31.54	54.71 ± 35.30
3	36.07 ± 31.67	35.90 ± 29.32	25.61 ± 21.71	42.58 ± 37.94
4	26.70 ± 29.14	23.36 ± 24.01	27.37 ± 31.45	36.83 ± 36.53
5	28.00 ± 29.40	16.09 ± 19.05	21.53 ± 27.29	25.23 ± 29.85
6	22.85 ± 25.52	12.78 ± 18.14	13.10 ± 21.02	15.95 ± 25.40
7	17.80 ± 22.86	4.61 ± 11.75	8.73 ± 15.09	15.18 ± 27.29
8	21.50 ± 29.35	4.39 ± 11.14**	4.25 ± 9.37**	9.23 ± 17.81*
9	13.70 ± 22.26	3.62 ± 10.49	6.00 ± 12.55	6.53 ± 13.03
10	10.75 ± 17.56	1.73 ± 8.38*	2.22 ± 7.49*	5.67 ± 12.00
11	16.57 ± 21.65	1.40 ± 6.93**	1.90 ± 6.17**	5.40 ± 11.54**

Note: Compared with the group of opium with buprenorphine, *$P < 0.05$, **$P < 0.01$.

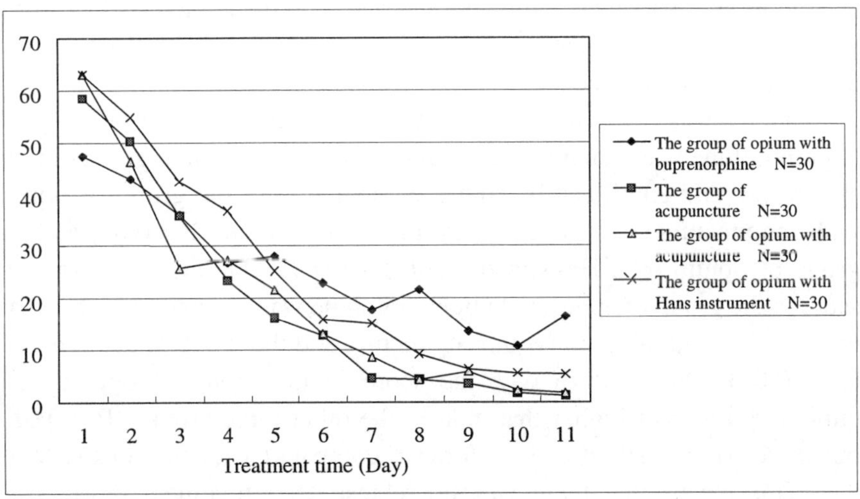

Figure 2.1. Visual Analogue Scale Craving Feelings (%).

2.3.4 *Statistics*

All data were analysed by the SPSS software. All quantitative data were showed by x ± SD.

2.4 Results

2.4.1

The effects of acupuncture in treating addicts on psycho-craving are shown in Table 2.1 and Fig. 2.1.

The craving feeling of the group of opium with buprenorphine was significantly higher than that of other groups on the eighth day (compared with the group of opium with acupuncture and the group of acupuncture $P < 0.01$; compared with the group of opium with Hans instrument $P < 0.05$). The craving feeling of the group of opium with buprenorphine was significantly higher than that of the group of opium with acupuncture and the group of acupuncture on the tenth day ($P < 0.05$). The craving feeling of the group of opium with buprenorphine was significantly higher than that of the other three groups on the 11th day ($P < 0.01$), while there was no significant difference compared with itself on the tenth day ($P > 0.05$), which indicated that there was no apparent relapse after all these four treatments were stopped.

The analysis revealed that the VAS score in the group of opium with buprenorphine was much higher than that in the other three groups in the eighth day and significantly higher compared with the group of opium with acupuncture ($P < 0.01$), the group of acupuncture ($P < 0.01$) and the group of opium with Hans instrument ($P < 0.05$). On the tenth day, the score in the group of opium with buprenorphine was apparently higher than that in the group of opium with acupuncture and the group of acupuncture ($P < 0.05$). On the 11th day, the score in the group of opium with buprenorphine was higher than that in the other three groups ($P < 0.01$), but there was no significant difference compared with that in the tenth day. This means that there was no relapse after treatment by all four methods.

2.5 Discussion

Craving has been described as a powerful urge to take drugs, and forces addicts to take drugs continuously or periodically to get psychological euphoria or avoid physical discomfort. It is a kind of psychological dependence caused by special euphoria and pleasure because of drug abuse. The level of craving for drugs is an index of psychological dependence.

Our research showed that on the eighth day, the level of craving was much higher in the group of opium with buprenorphine than that in the other three groups. Similar results were observed on the 11th day. On the tenth day, the craving in the group of opium with buprenorphine was apparently higher than that in the group of opium with acupuncture and the group of acupuncture. That means acupuncture with or without Hans instrument had better effects on suppressing the craving for heroin than opium with buprenorphine. The results indicated that acupuncture might be a perspective alternative in treating the psychological dependence in the later period of de-addiction.

Most researchers believe that heroin produces euphoria or pleasurable feelings and can be a positive reinforcer by interacting with the reward pathway in the brain, which is the reason of psychological dependence. It is known that there are many areas within the dopaminergic reward pathway in the central nervous system (CNS), which include arcuate nucleus, amygdaloid nucleus, locus ceruleus, grey matter around centre canal, the ventral tegmental area (VTA) and nucleus accumbens. The VTA and nucleus accumbens are considered as the final pathway of the reward effects caused by addictive drugs. Opiate drugs can cause both direct and indirect reward pathway. Some studies (Tang and Li, 1999) show that D1 receptors in the system of reward pathway with DA may attribute to the euphoria related to sensation, while D2 receptors in the DA systems of VTA and marginal forebrain attribute to the euphoria related to craving for drugs. Research of brain imaging show that the excitation of midbrain-margin DA circuit is the nervous basis for euphoria (Yan and Wei, 1998). The frontal and temporal lobes attend the memorial procedure of addictive behaviors. The main reasons for psychological dependence and craving are extreme euphoria and the memory of euphoria. Acupuncture may suppress the craving by suppressing the excitation of midbrain-margin DA circuit, frontal and temporal lobes. But this conclusion needs to be further proven by brain imaging.

References

Ge, Y., Li, M. and Zheng, J.W. (1995) Clinical assessment on potential analgesics dependence. *Chin. J. Drug Depend.* **4**(2), 73–74.

Tang, Y.L. and Li, J. (1999) Research of prevention and treatment and nervous mechanism on heroin dependence. *Chin. J. Drug Depend.* **8**(2), 151–154.

Yan, Z. and Wei, F. (1998) Application of modern brain imaging on addiction research. *Chin. J. Drug Depend.* **7**(2), 65–69.

Zhang, S.C. (1997) Speech on the Academic Conference of National Research on Prevention and Treatment of Drug Dependence and Drug Abuse. *Chin. Bull. Drug Depend.* **6**(3), 129.

Chapter 3

Advances in Research of Angiogenesis Effect of Traditional Chinese Medicine

Zhi-shan Ding & Xing-de Yuo

Abstract

Angiogenesis is a cruxial phenomenon in the balance of physiological metabolic processes. In the situations of pathological changes, very often, imbalanced angiogenesis is observed: over-activity leads to over-growth, whereas under-activity is responsible for necrosis and fibrosis. Disease-related angiogenesis occurs in tumours, diabetic retinal lesions, rheumatoid arthritis, etc. On the other hand, defective angiogenesis occurs in ulcerations, bone necrosis and fibrosis. Chinese medicine has been known to possess anti-angiogenic effects in animal experiments. Tripterygium wilfordic selectively inhibited the proliferation of vascular endothelial cells. Anti-cancer formulae have been found to control the growth of cancer cell cultures. On the other hand, Chinese medicinal herbs and formulae supporting circulation and Qi, are also plentiful. It is therefore suggested that research on Chinese medicine can concentrate more on angiogenesis.

Keywords: Chinese Medicine; Angiogenesis.

3.1 Introduction

Angiogenesis refers to the budding and growth of a new vascular system from an existing vascular bed. In recent years, this has become a hot topic in bioscience research. Recent research revealed that angiogenesis plays an important role in physiologic and pathologic processes and is strictly regulated by a balance between positive and negative regulatory signals. If the balance is lost, disease related to angiogenesis can result (Carmeliet and Jain, 2000). Such diseases include tumours, diabetic retinal lesions, rheumatic arthritics, psoriasis, angioma and atherosclerosis, which have persistent vascular growth. Basically, these are diseases that do great harm to people's health. However, defective angiogenesis cannot provide a good response, like healing of trauma, ulceration, bone injury or microcirculatory defects and it can directly affect the treatment of disease. Traditional Chinese Medicine (TCM) therapy has a long history of relationship with diseases concerning angiogenesis. It is different from western medicine in character, and is superior in the treatment of these diseases. Therefore, the development of new TCM drugs to promote angiogenesis has great significance in the elucidation of basic principles, clinical treatment and in the field of TCM drug research.

3.2 Angiogenesis and Disease

No tissues and cells in the human body can exist and proliferate without blood vessels which supply nutrient substance and discharge metabolic products. Angiogenesis is a biological process which involves the growth of new blood vessels on the base of a pre-existing vascular bed, and is the result of the interaction of cells, matrix and cell factors. In mature organs, the blood vessels are in its grown-up form and its endothelium is in a state of rest and non-proliferation. The formation of normal vascular network appears in cyclic changes of female genital organs and in developing embryos and they are under strict control. But new angiogenesis can also appear in pathologic conditions like trauma, tumours, rheumatic arthritic psoriasis and atherosclerosis. In 1987, Folkman called diseases with this kind of abnormal capillary proliferation "angiogenetic disease". In accordance with different effects on angiogenesis, two kinds of treatment have been established. One kind is called therapeutic angiogenesis, which causes the increase of capillaries and the enhancement of blood flow, by the use of drugs or genetic transformation to promote cardiac capillary angiogenesis for the relief of myocardial ischemic symptoms (Durairaj *et al.*, 2000). Another is termed therapeutic anti-angiogenesis which refers to the inhibition of abnormal capillary proliferation to attain curative effect, by the use of drugs to counteract tumour angiogenesis so that it reaches a state that can be cured (Ryan and Wilding, 2000). At present, these two methods have been applied clinically and have attained comparatively ideal results.

3.2.1 *Angiogenesis and tumours*

Primary tumour growth, and metastasis all depend on the existing blood vessels and new angiogenesis, and they establish their own blood supply system from the matrix of the host. More and more studies demonstrate that angiogenesis is very important in the growth and metastasis of solid tumours. At the pre-metastatic stage, there is a marked enhancement of angiogenesis, the degree of which is in positive correlation with the metastasising ability of the tumour. This shows that tumour tissue must get nutritional supply from the host in order to develop local growth. Therefore, the stoppage of angiogenesis and interruption of the path of nutritional supply of the tumour have become new objectives in anti-tumour treatment. Researchers are now putting emphasis on the research of drugs for destruction or inhibition of angiogenesis and for effective interruption of tumour growth and metastasis. This kind of drugs are called tumour angiogenesis inhibitors, which can be divided into two major categories. The first category consists of specific inhibitors which can specifically inhibit vascular endothelial cell proliferation but exert no inhibitory effect on tumour cells. Examples include vasoinhibitor, TNP-470, etc. The second category consists of non-specific inhibitors, which have inhibitory effects on vascular endothelial cells as well as tumour cells. Examples include suramin, interleukin, etc. In the early 1970s, Folkman raised the idea of using anti-angiogenesis therapy to treat tumours. Now, it has become an important area in the field of tumour therapy and prevention in investigating the mechanism of angiogenesis and the discovery of effective angiogenesis inhibitors.

3.2.2 *Angiogenesis and atherosclerosis*

Atherosclerosis is the most common cause of many kinds of acute and chronic cardiovascular diseases. The atherosclerotic plaques may cause the narrowing of the vascular lumen or may even be detached to cause obstruction and arterial spasm, which may lead to tissue ischemia, hypoxia and cellular damage. Therefore, interruption or regression of the development of atherosclerosis is a basic approach in the treatment of various acute cardiocerebral conditions.

Atherosclerosis is a long term process — it is generally considered that the chief causes are the increase of plasma low density lipoprotein, migration of mononuclear large phagocytes and proliferation of smooth muscle cells. From the production and development of atherosclerosis, it can be seen that under effective control of thrombus formation, atherosclerosis is a comparatively benign chronic disease that is similar to benign tumour, and it is only when the atherosclerotic plaque obstructs the vessel or cracks to form thrombus that life might be jeopardized. The normal coronary artery wall has no capillaries, but in the development of atherosclerotic plaque, capillaries grow inside the plaque for the transportation of nutrients to the smooth muscle cells and large phagocytes within to form a compact capillary network — vasa vasorum. The intravascular nutritional channels have some fragile vessels which may be easily injured by lipid peroxide inside the plaque and bleed, and this may trigger the formation of thrombus, leading to tissue ischemia and hypoxia. Therefore, angiogenesis plays an important role in the formation and development of atherosclerotic plaque.

In March 1999, Folkmam *et al.* used the anti-angiogenesis drug TNP-40 to treat atherosclerosis in rats with deficient Apoprotein E (Apo E) and demonstrated with certainty that anti-atherosclerosis can cause regression of atherosclerosis and that angiogenesis can promote the development of the plaque. Similar to atherosclerosis, tumours are caused by abnormal proliferation of cells and are also associated with abnormal vascular proliferation (Zhu *et al.*, 2000).

3.2.3 *Angiogenesis and rheumatoid arthritis*

In the early stage of rheumatoid arthritis, the pathological changes are persistent synovitis and pannus formation, which are especially dependent on the widely existing new vascular network. The pannus has characteristics similar to tumour tissue — it can invade the joint cartilage and bone tissue, leading to the loss of joint function. Clinical studies demonstrated that the degree of intra-articular new vascular proliferation of rheumatoid arthritis is proportional to the severity of disease and the degree of synovial hyperplasia. The formation of new blood vessels in rheumatoid arthritis is divided into three steps: the activation of endothelial cells by inflammatory medium; the degradation of vascular endothelial matrix by proteinase; and endothelial cell migration and formation of new blood vessels. Animal experimentations demonstrated that effective inhibition of formation of new blood vessels of the pannus can relieve experimental arthritis — this provides a new approach to the clinical treatment and prevention of rheumatoid arthritis.

3.3 Factors Affecting Angiogenesis

Angiogenesis involves wide interaction among cells, soluble factors and extracellular ingredients. Endothelial cells receive the required information of establishing vascular network through four different steps: (1) proteinase causing dissolution of matrix membrane; (2) migration of endothelial cells; (3) proliferation of endothelial cells; and (4) formation of capillary blood vessels. Angiogenesis is influenced and controlled by corrected cytopoiesis factors produced by various kinds of cells, involving cells like mononuclear large phagocytes, lymphocytes mastocytes, tumour cells and endothelial cells. At present, at least 20 kinds of cell-activating factors like vaso-endothelial growth factor (VEGF), acid fibroblast growth factor (aFGF) and alkaline fibroblast growth factor (bFGF) have been found. Through *in vitro* and animal experiments, ten more effective angiogenesis inhibitors have been found, some of which include angiostatin, endostatin, TNP-470, etc.

3.4 TCM and Angiogenesis

Treatment of angiogenesis diseases with TCM has marked effectiveness. Treatment of this kind of disease through anti-angiogenesis may be due to one of the cellular and molecular mechanisms. This explains why TCM can treat different diseases with the same drugs. Research on the character of TCM drugs in promoting angiogenesis and anti-angiogenesis has become popular, especially studies concerning tumour treatment with anti-angiogenesis drugs. Some anti-angiogenesis components have been separated, like radix ginseng saponin Rg3, tripterine of tripterygium wilfordii, etc.

3.4.1 *Anti-angiogenetic TCM drugs*

Tripterygium wilfordic has a definite effect on angiogenetic diseases like rheumatoid arthritis, tumour, psoriasis and atherosclerosis. This suggests that tripterygium wilfordic may have anti-angiogenesis effect. Ju Jin Bo *et al.* used 5 g/ml tripterygium wilfordin to act on the vascular endothelial cells of mice and the result showed that triptergium wilfordin can inhibit the migration and proliferation of vascular endothelial cells, and can also promote the synthesis of extracellular matrix and inhibit the activity of integrin. Therefore, tripterygium wilfordii can control the angiogenesis process through various mechanisms (Zhu *et al.*, 1996a). Ju Jin Bo *et al.* observed the influence of Fu Tai Bao (a TCM compound agent containing tripterygium wilfordii) on the biological activity of vascular endothelial cells and its therapeutic mechanism on the treatment of psoriasis. The result showed that Fu Tai Bao can inhibit vascular endothelial cell migration into vascular lumen, promote vascular endothelial cells to synthesise extra-cellular matrix type IV collagen protein, fibrin-linked protein and matrix membrane-linked protein, regulate the expression of integrin and increase significantly the activity of calcium-dependent adhesion ingredients. All these suggest that Fu Tai Bao can regulate and control the process of angiogenesis through various mechanisms (Zhu *et al.*, 1996b). Gao Yong *et al.* used the monomer tripterine extracted from tripterygium wilfordii for the study of anti-angiogenesis activity and the result showed that 0.1 mg/ml tripterine can completely inhibit tubulc formation ability of human venous endothelial cells stimulated by tumour cell culture medium solution, and 0.01 mg/ml cavity-tripterine can markedly inhibit the growth of endothelial cells (Gao *et al.*, 1998). Chun Xi Jong *et al.* used different vascular endothelial cell strains to conduct similar experiments and obtained the same result — that tripterine had an anti-angiogenesis effect (Chen *et al.*, 1999).

Yan Da Hai *et al.* used chicken embryo in a screening study of 43 anti-carcinoma formulas and selected 13 drugs which appeared most frequently in anti-angiogenesis investigation, and the result was that rhizoma zedoariae and radix curcumae had an anti-angiogenesis effect (Yan *et al.*, 1998). The experiments performed by Juang Xie Ling demonstrated that semen coicis injection had an anti-angiogenesis effect (Jiang *et al.*, 2000). The research of Shu Jong Ping *et al.* showed that thallus eckloniae polysaccharide sulfate can inhibit the formation of tubular structure by endothelial cells and also vascular formation by chicken embryo chorionic allantoid membrane and possesses anti-growth activity to RIF-1 rat tumour. It is an inhibitor of the adhesion of alkaline fibroblast growth factor (bFGF) and of the proliferation of bFGF-dependent cells (Xu *et al.*, 1999). Mon Yin Chai used the rabbit cornea alkaline burning model for investigation and demonstrated that compound radix salviae miltiorrhizae injection could inhibit formation of new growing vessels in the alkaline burn cornea, showing that compound radix salviae miltiorrhizae injection had an anti-angiogenesis effect (Meng *et al.*, 1995). Many epidemiologic studies show that tea drinking can lower the risk of gastrointestinal tumours, esophageal carcinoma, lung cancer, and inhibit angiogenesis (Wang, 2000). Bufalin is one of the brifogenin components in sceretis bufonis; it not only induces apoptosis of tumour cells, it can also inhibit angiogenesis (Xu *et al.*, 2000).

Rhizome curcumae longae is a TCM drug used to activate blood circulation and remove stasis and is a common component in the anti-tumour formula. Its chief acting ingredient, curcumin, is especially effective in tumour treatment. We used the chicken embryo chorionic allantois model and tumour cell culture strains to observe the effect of rhizoma curcumae longae on angiogenesis, and found that it could significantly inhibit angiogenesis in the chicken embryo chorionic allantoid membrane (Ding *et al.*, 2003). Shen Mai injection originates from the formula Shen Mai San mentioned in the book "Qian Jin Yao Fang" and is a derivative formula of Shen Mai San, which is composed of radix ginseng and radix ophiopogonis, being effective in replenishing vital energy and nourishing Yin. Our study revealed that Shen Mai injection can significantly inhibit the proliferation of cow endothelial cells in cow plasma and tumour culture broth, but had no apparent inhibitory effect on non-endothelial cells including tumour cells and smooth muscle cells. Shen Mai injection can significantly inhibit cow endothelial cell migration in cow plasma culture broth and tumour culture broth. It can also inhibit tumour growth, decrease capillary density in tumour hot spot area and decrease the expression of bFGF, MMP-2 and PCNA in tumour tissue. Therefore, Shen Mai is considered a specific inhibitor of angiogenesis (Yi *et al.*, 2002).

3.4.2 *TCM promotion of angiogenesis*

Promotion of angiogenesis through genetic transformation has undergone clinical investigation. In particular, the treatment of myocardial ischemia in coronary disease has evoked general attention. TCM considers that "*qi* and blood are correlated", "if *qi* can pass through, the circulation is smooth", "supplement *qi* and activate blood", "the circulation is the residence of blood". So TCM drugs that have the characteristics of activating vital energy and blood circulation are effective in promotion of angiogenesis. This provides theoretical basis of angiogenesis effect of TCM drugs and its application has already been used (Wang and Wu, 2000; Dai and Li, 2000).

Zhang Shu Cheng *et al.* used the chicken embryo allaniod membrane angiogenesis model to investigate the angiogenesis effect of drugs for kidney tonic and haemopoiesis and regulation of menstruation in animal serum. The result showed that the two kinds of TCM drugs had specific angiogenesis effect: they could promote significantly angiogenesis, increase the number of blood vessels ($P < 0.01$) and there was an increase of 55%–124% in angiogenesis promotion. Zhang Shu Cheng *et al.* used old female gold colour hamster for the animal study (coincide with senile physiologic weakness of kidney symptoms) of morphologic pharmacology of two kinds of TCM drugs. They discovered that angiogenesis in uterine tissue increased markedly and considered that the angiogenesis effect of TCM drugs was of much significance (Zhang *et al.*, 1998 and 2000b). Radix astragalic is commonly used to treat chronic dermal ulceration and unhealed traumatic lesions. Zhu Jin Bo *et al.* used endothelial cell strains for study and found that radix astragali had better angiogenesis promotion effect and this might be the important mechanism of its effectiveness on chronic dermal ulceration (Zhu *et al.*, 1996).

Wang Wei Jia *et al.* used the rabbit bone fracture model for research and found that TCM for tonification of kidney and activation of circulation can shorten the time of organisation of haematoma, promote the proliferation of local vascular endothelial cells and fibroblasts and regeneration of capillaries and shorten the healing process of bone fracture (Wang *et al.*, 1998). Zhang Jian Guo *et al.* used both tibia of a rabbit to make a fracture model and wrapped it with a TCM paste outside (which consist of Resina boswelliae cartevii, commiphora myrrha, flos carthami, resina thraconis, radix notoginseng, etc.). It was revealed that TCM drugs could promote vasodilatation, vascular regeneration and increase blood supply to the fracture area and blood vessel. Regenerations in the study group was faster than in the control group. The result suggests that TCM drugs can accelerate the vascular developing process of fracture site and ensure the blood supply in the process of healing to promote recovery of bone fracture (Zhang *et al.*, 2000a).

3.5 Conclusion

The research of TCM drugs from the viewpoint of angiogenesis is a comparatively late development, and this may be due to the insufficient understanding of angiogenesis from the perspective of TCM. If deeper investigation, using TCM principles, can be conducted to reveal the relation between angiogenesis and diseases, the research of treating angiogenetic disease with TCM will be further developed. The significance is that the continuous improvement of angiogenesis research, in principles and methodologies, would enhance TCM drug development on angiogenesis-related diseases. This will in turn lead to the modernisation of Traditional Chinese Medicine.

References

Carmeliet, P. and Jain, R.K. (2000) Angiogenesis in cancer and other diseases. *Nature* **407**(6801), 249–257.

Chen, S.-Z., Ji, L., Wang, Y.-P. *et al.* (1999) *In vitro* study of red pigment in killing liver endothelial cells of mice. *Qien Wei J. Med. Pharm.* **16**(6), 337–339.

Dai, R.-H. and Li, Y. (2000) Curative angiogenesis of myocardial infarction and traditional Chinese medicine. *Chin. J. Integr. Tradit. West. Med.* **20**(3), 163–164.

Ding, C.-S., Gao, C.-X., Chen, N.-B. *et al.* (2003) Effects of curcumin: anti-angiogenesis and induction of SMMC-7721 cell apoptosis. *Chin. Pharm. Sci.* **19**(2), 171–173.

Durairaj, A., Mehra, A., Singh, R.P., *et al.* (2000) Therapeutic angiogenesis. *Cardiol. Rev.* **8**(5), 279–287.

Gao, Y., Wang, J.-J., Mei, C.-L. *et al.* (1998) Experimental study of red pigment in depressing of vascular growth. *Tumor* **18**(4), 280–281.

Jiang, X.-L., Zhang, L., Xu, C.-Y. *et al.* (2000) The effect of Coicis Semen Injection on angiogenesis. *Tumor* **20**(4), 313–314.

Meng, X., Wang, J. and Qi, L.-P. (1995) Study of compound injection of Danshen in inhibiting angiogenesis in post-alkali burned corneas. *China J. Ophthal. Tradit. Chin. Med.* **5**(4), 195–197.

Ryan, C.J. and Wilding, G. (2000) Angiogenesis inhibitors: new agents in cancer therapy. *Drugs Aging* **17**(4), 249–255.

Wang, L. and Wu, C.-K. (2000) Recent advances of angiogenesis enhancing activity in clinical application. *Shenzhen J. Integr. Tradit. West. Med.* **10**(3), 130–133.

Wang, W.-J., Xu, L.-W. and Yu, H.-P. (1998) Experimental study of tonifying kidney and promoting blood TCM on bone fracture healing. *Chin. J. Basic Med. Tradit. Chin. Med.* **4**(9), 35–38.

Wang, Z.-L. (2000) Tea drink and inhibition of angiogenesis. *Foreign Med. Sci. (Sect. Hyg.)* **27**(3), 190.

Xu, R.-C., Chen, X.-Y. and Chen, L. (2000) Recent advances of Bufalin anti-cancer mechanic. *Foreign Med. Sci. (Oncol. Sect.)* **27**(4), 202–204.

Xu, Z.-P., Li, F.-C. and Wang, H.-R. (1999) The effect of Laminarin sulphate in inhibiting of angiogenesis and anti-tumor activity. *Chin. Tradit. Herb. Drug* **30**(7), 551–553.

Yan, D.-H., Zhu, S.-H. and Fu, Z.-B. (1998) Screening herbs of inhibiting angiogenesis growth with click chorioallantoic membrane assay. *Heilongjiang J. Med. Pharm.* **11**(2), 94.

Yi, L.-H., Diang, C.-S., Gao, C.-X. *et al.* (2002) Experimental study on effect of angiogenesis with Shenmai Injection. *Chin. J. Integr. Tradit. West. Med.* **22**(10), 761–763.

Zhang, J.-G., Chen, L.-J. and Jiang, W.-Y. (2000a) Effect of external application of Chinese medicinal herbs on reconstruction of micrangium in fracture healing. *China J. Orthop. Trauma* **13**(2), 86–87.

Zhang, S.-C., Wu, C.-K. and Shan, M.-S. (1998) Effect of prescription of tonifying kidney to regulate menstruation and Bu Shen Sheng Xue on improvement of angiogenesis. *Chin. J. Basic Med. Tradit. Chin. Med.* **4**(8), 37–38.

Zhang, S.-C., Wu, C.-K., Wang, L. *et al.* (2000b) Experimental study of Bu Shen Sheng Xue and Bu Shen Tiao Jin TCM in angiogenesis. *J. Tradit. Chin. Med.* **41**(6), 369–370.

Zhu, J.-J., Geo, W. and Chen, G.-H. (2000) Effect of edostatin in tumor growth and atherosclerosis formation. *Progr. Physiol. Sci.* **31**(3), 243–245.

Zhu, J.-B. *et al.* (1996a) The effects of Tripterygium on biological activity of vascular endothelial cells. *China J. Tradit. Chin. Med. Sci.* **3**(1), 16–18.

Zhu, J.-B. *et al.* (1996b) The effects of herbal mixture contained Radix Salvia Miltiorrhiza and Zicao (*Arnebia* sp) on biological activity of mice vascular endothelial cells. *Chin. J. Dermatol.* **29**(4), 249–251.

Zhu, J.-B., Li, Y.-D. and Li, Y.-S. (1996c) Mechanism of Huang Qi improving angiogenesis during treatment of chronic skin ulcer. *Hebei J. Tradit. Chin. Med.* **18**(4), 21–22.

Chapter 4

The Rationale of Combination Drug Formulas in Traditional Chinese Medicine

Jie Wang, Lin-guo Zhang & Wei Jia

Abstract

The following points are addressed in this paper through the discussion of combination formula research. (1) The study of combination formulas should follow the TCM theory and principle of drug compatibility, pure chemistry or chemical isolates-oriented research should be avoided. (2) The study of combination formula of TCM should actively explore the unknown physiological and pathological mechanisms as well as the preventive and treatment methodology of diseases. (3) The study of pharmacologically active ingredients from combination formula may facilitate an overall improvement of TCM research. (4) A combination formula should be regarded as a whole during the research. (5) The pharmacological study of combination formula investigates the principle and rationale of drug combination and compatibility, and will help ascertain the mechanism of action and therapeutic substances in the formulas. (6) It is necessary to study pharmacokinetics of TCM although it is technically challenging. (7) Multidisciplinary approach should be taken during the research of combination formulas. (8) Clinical efficacy is the scientific basis of research with combination formulas.

Keywords: Combination Formulas; Traditional Chinese Medicine; TCM Theory.

4.1 Introduction

The combination drug formulas in traditional Chinese medicine (TCM) consist of ancient prescriptions, which have been proven effective through thousands of years of clinical practice, as well as the newly developed formulas based on clinical experience over the past several decades. With the inception, growth and development of TCM, the combination drug formulas have experienced a long development process, and thus far have become the main treatment modality in today's traditional medicine in China. A good formula is not simply a pile-up of medicinal herbs, the selection of individual drugs in the formula is guided by traditional medical theory and contemplations, and strictly follows the rules of drug combination and compatibility. Today, with the rapid development of modern science and information technology and the use of multi-disciplinary approach in medical society, the study of combination drug formulas needs to absorb different knowledge and perspectives and move forward while inheriting the traditional experience, thoughts and theories. This paper discusses issues involved in the research of combination drug formulas and our personal understanding of this field.

4.2 The Study of Combination Drug Formulas and TCM

Before the 17th century, Western traditional science was based on structuralism, and characterised by the laws of public-acknowledged truth. This was different from the framework of modern Western scientific system, which stresses on analysis and evidence. The traditional Chinese science was based on the "theory of birth-to-death" and characterised by the cycle-production model. Influenced by the thinking model of traditional culture, TCM takes Qi as its core conception to describe and summarise the live activities of the human body, and uses Yin and Yang and the Five Elements as its basic model to establish a system of physiology, pathology, diagnosis and therapy of diseases. Although it has not reached the quantitative level of modern medicine in the respect of biological analysis, it describes the life regulation with different perspectives, including society, culture, physiology and psychology. In this regard, TCM views life and life phenomenon as a whole and in a dynamic way, which appears to be superior to our modern medical science.

Medicine and herbs are indispensable. Certain medicine brings certain herbs. For centuries, Chinese herbs have been used to prevent and cure diseases under the guidance of the TCM theory. The combination drug formulas have different pharmacological and therapeutic principles from the Western pharmaceuticals and compounding formulas based on Western theory of disease prevention and treatment. The rationale of the combination drug formula reflects the TCM concept which views the body as a whole, and views a disease dialectically, while the selection of herbs reflects the principle of quality, tastes, channels of distribution, and laws of drug combination and compatibility in a formula. Combining basic TCM theory with research on ancient, empirical and contemporary formulas may generate new perspectives with scientific significance, this is also where the advantage of combination formula in clinical and basic research lies. Dialectics and other philosophical ideas can be found in every part of TCM, and TCM also stresses the dynamic physiological and pathological changes in organs, blood, Qi and Yin-Yang. Any change in a TCM drug formula will alter the chemical ingredients, and in result, affect the clinical efficacy. This indicates that the research of formula cannot break away from the "track" of basic TCM theory.

The difference between a single-herb formula and a simple combination formula consisting of two herbs is not merely an addition of more herbs, but also the interaction between the herbal drugs. A system of extensive interaction and inter-relation among herbal drugs is formed in a relatively big, multi-herb formula. A combination drug formula does not mean a quantitative addition of different herbs but more complex interaction and inter-relationship among herbs with different therapeutic functions. The human body is an open and complex system composed of various physiological and pathological factors. In a view of systematic science, nature is a macroscopic system in which lives and substances are inter related, a combination formula containing natural plants and animal parts is actually inseparable from the human body, and therefore, it becomes possible that such a formula could restore the balance of an imbalanced human body (Zhang, 2000a).

Recently, much progress has been made in the study of traditional combination formula with modern chemical pharmacological technology, but most of the results explain the clinical efficacy and mechanism by means of known biological parameters in modern medicine (such as molecules, cells, tissues, organs, etc.). It has not taken into account the unknown physiological and pathological mechanisms of a known disease.

In this regard, the TCM which rationally combines the disease symptoms, therapeutic methodology, combination formulas and treatment effectiveness may hold the potential for further development towards the most reliable medical theory.

4.3 The Study of Chemical Ingredients in Combination Formulas

The development of a new chemical drug (NCE), generally starting from chemical synthesis, relies greatly on the structural analysis and characterisation of physiochemical properties of the compound. A combination formula, on the other hand, contains a group of phytochemicals, in which a cooperative action of chemical ingredients such as polysaccharides, polypeptides, proteins, and other molecules plays a fundamental role in the treatment of diseases. It has been proven by years of practice that research of formula and herbs should stress on finding the effective ingredients. The use of modern research means to identify effective ingredients from a combination formula would enrich the pharmacology of TCM, promote the overall TCM research, and hopefully, enhance the clinical efficacy.

The overall effect of a combination formula is not merely the quantitative addition or summation of the effect of each herb used in the formula. And the chemical ingredients in a formula are not presented simply by a summation of the ingredients in each herb. The aim of research with combination formula is to pursue the best overall therapeutic effect, while understanding of individual isolates and chemical extracts of a formula is also important. Two important questions should be stressed here: firstly, how to ascertain the effective ingredients in a combination formula? We believe that the formula can be regarded as a whole, ingredients that have similar chemical properties can be separated into groups such as saponin, flavone and alkaloid, etc. If certain chemical ingredients contained in a group play major therapeutic roles based on pharmacological studies in animal models, the group in the formula can be regarded as an active group. Hundreds of ingredients from combination formulas can be divided into about ten groups, with each containing tens of ingredients confirmed by means of modern separation and analytical methods. Secondly, how to combine the research of active ingredients with the rationalisation of combination formulas? We can use one or two active compounds in each individual herb in a combination formula as quantitative and qualitative standard(s) or indicator(s), and compare their pharmacology and pharmacodynamics individually and combined as a whole. Through extensive studies *in vitro*, *in vivo*, and in cell and molecular biology levels we ascertain the active compounds and groups, understand the mechanism of action, and rationalise the combination and compatibility of a specific herbal formula.

During the decoction process of formula, many physical and chemical changes will occur in herbal ingredients. For example, the change of pH may change content of certain chemical ingredients, and therefore, may alter the effectiveness of the formula. It also requires in-depth research on how to define the coherence of chemical ingredients from one herb to formula, how they function on each other, and whether there are new compounds generated through such a decoction process? For example, it was found in the study of a formula, "Liu-Wei-Di-Huang", that the chemical ingredients in the decoction were no longer the same as the sum of all herbs participated in the formula. New peaks were found in thin-layer chromatography (TLC) scanning, indicating the generation of new components. Although progress has been made in this respect, many questions remain unanswered. Conclusions should not be drawn at this stage as to whether new components are significant in the treatment and whether those so-called "non-active" components can be defined as "non-active" with the current pharmacological means.

Results from pharmacological studies of the active ingredients in a combination formula may not match the description in traditional theory, although we believe the study of combination formulas should follow the TCM theory. It is likely that the research of chemical ingredients of the formula may discover or generate new compounds or new drugs, or new opinions, but a tendency or focus on going "all the way" to chemical isolates in the research of the combination formula should be avoided. To develop a new phytomedicine with known active isolates or groups extracted from herbs is a different approach from the traditional formula, although it is viewed as a new addition of modern TCM development.

4.4 Pharmacological Study with Regard to the Rationale and Compatibility of Different Herbal Drugs Selected in a Combination Formula

To summarise and rationalise the compounding of the traditional herbal formulas is perhaps the most important part of pharmacological research of combination formulas. It can help ascertain the pharmaceutical substances in a formula, understand the mechanism of action, and facilitate the safe and effective use of TCM agents. Great progress has been made in TCM pharmacology with the development of serum-TCM pharmacology, compound-TCM pharmacology, TCM-isolates pharmacology, etc. in recent years.

The pharmacological study of combination drug formula mainly involves following four aspects (Zhang, 2000a and b).

(1) The study of herbal interactions showed that there are different forms of inter-relationships between herbal drugs in a well-organised formula; such as synergism (two drugs with similar effect reinforcing each other), assisting (strengthening effect of another drug), detoxication, antagonism (reducing curative effects) and rejection (increasing toxicity). The research with "Sini Decoction", a well-known combination formula, showed that this compounding agent could significantly strengthen myocardium. One of the herbal drugs in this formula, Aconite Root (*Radix aconiti Praeparata*), has a mild effect of strengthening the heart. However, when combined with Dried Ginger (*Rhizoma Zingiberis*) in the formula, it can readily increase the contraction of myocardium, dilate the coronary artery, which is the evidence of relationship of drug reinforcement. Additionally, the combined use of these two herbal drugs, Aconite Root and Dried Ginger, greatly reduced the toxicity as observed individually. So the relationship between Aconite Root and Dried Ginger in the formula is "synergism" and "detoxication".

(2) The research with combination drug formulas indicated that the proper use of dosage and ratio/proportion of different herbs in the formula is of key importance in obtaining a satisfactory efficacy. The research of "Decoction of Peony and Liquorice"

showed that the best ratio of Peony Root (*Radix paeoniae rubra*) and Liquorice (*Radix glycyrrhizae*) was 2:1, which resulted in the best pain-relief effect.

(3) Study the compatibility of herbs in a formula based on TCM theory, which includes four natures and five flavours, channel tropism, effects of lifting, lowering, floating and sinking. Research into the "Hua-tuo Pill" discovered that borneol in the formula facilitated the penetration of one of the alkaloids (namely, tetramethylpyrazine) of *Rhizoma ligustici chuanxiong* across the blood-brain barrier, and significantly increased the concentration of the alkaloids in brain. This is a clear example of "channel tropism" in TCM.

(4) Research on serum pharmacology of a single herb formula and a combination formula has been carried out by a number of investigators. The serum was collected at different time points after the administration of combination formulas and tested *in vitro*. This would, to some extent, match the drug metabolism and pharmacological activities *in vivo* (Zhang, 2000b).

Any change in herbs and dosage in a formula will greatly alter the pharmacokinetics of the drug. Traditional formulas are mostly administered orally, and the chemical ingredients will change in the gastrointestinal tract through decomposition, hydrolysis and other metabolising processes. Such an important chemical change *in vivo* may play a vital role in disease treatment. The development of science, starting from its early stages with little knowledge of the nature, gradually transforming into a comprehensive and multi-disciplinary theory, is a long process of continuous practice and self-improvement. Similarly, the development of TCM is also a process of integrating philosophy, Confucianism, Taoism, astronomy, and other thoughts accumulating over 5000 years. The further development of TCM demands continuous absorption of the multidisciplinary subjects and technological achievements in modern science. Fortunately, new research methodologies and hypotheses such as "the cumulative measurement of herbal drugs," "the pharmacokinetics of active components in combination formula," "serum pharmacology," etc. have been adopted and have significantly facilitated the development of combination formula research.

4.5 Issues on the Participation of Multidisciplines

One of the most important characteristics with modern science is multi-disciplinary approach. In the investigation of compatibility of all herbal components in combination formulas, it is a general practice to use animal models of various kinds to observe pharmacological effectiveness. Thus, modern animal experimentation has become an important part of TCM research, as well as TCM modernisation. Due to the fact that there are many ambiguous expressions, conceptual and theoretical explanations and empirical methodologies existing in TCM, it is important to use mathematical and computational technology to perform quantitative research, and thus, break the limitation of such a traditional field. It is also essential to apply pharmaceutical chemistry, analytical chemistry, technology of modern pharmaceutics, molecular spectrometers, chromatography, x-ray diffraction, etc. in basic research on combination formulas. The mechanism of how a combination formula modulates the gene groups is not known. The latest technology such as *in situ*, live and real-time detection, micro-section, micro-dialysis, molecular radar, as well as drug screening technology built on cell and molecular levels can enhance the success rate of active substance identification from a proven formula.

In the meantime, the modern chemical and engineering technology such as super-critical fluid extraction, preparation chromatography, etc. can be used to solve the key problems of separation, condensation and formation of herbal extracts on a large scale.

4.6 Prospects

Research on combination formula is a complex systems engineering process. Clinical efficacy is and should be the scientific basis of the study of formula. The main function and compatibility of all herbs in combination formulas are the prerequisites of the study. And the work involving differentiation, optimisation, selection of combination formulas, use of appropriate pharmacological models and multidisciplinary technology would be the main avenue of establishing TCM chemistry and pharmacology. A different avenue of developing modern phytomedicine can be established through careful selection, separation and extraction of chemical constituents with important therapeutic effectiveness from combination formulas. With the emergence of new technology and research findings, the TCM foundation of our ancestors should be supplemented, revised and further developed, which not only coincides with the general law of scientific development, but also benefits the modernisation of TCM industry.

References

Zhang, S. P. (2000a) Research of drug substances with combination formulas of TCM, *Chin. J. Basic Med. TCM* **6**(6), 56.

Zhang, S. T. (2000b) Advances in pharmacokinetics of combination formulas of TCM, *J. An-hui TCM College* **19**(3), 58.

chemical constituents with increasing the therapeutic effectiveness from combination formulas. With the emergence of new technology and research findings, the TCM formulation theories should be supplemented, [illegible] and further developed, [illegible] [illegible] developments [illegible] [illegible] medicine [illegible] formulas.

References

Wang, X. [illegible] (19[illegible]) [illegible] [illegible] combination [illegible]. [illegible] [illegible]
Zhang, [illegible] [illegible] [illegible] [illegible] [illegible]. [illegible] 19[illegible].

Chapter 5

Approaches in Treating AIDS with Chinese Medicine

Wei-bo Lu

Abstract

Chinese medicine has been used in China as an adjuvant therapy in the treatment of AIDS. Unlike modern therapeutic treatment which applies a reductional approach, using directly targeting drugs and their combination, Chinese medicine applies a holistic direction. The holistic approach is aimed at the internal balance of vital forces, which achieves good harmony when the individual is healthy. AIDS patients suffer from a severe loss of ability to maintain the vital forces at an equilibrium. Immuno-enhancement should be the key. Indeed many herbs and herbal formulae are commonly known to be rich in immuno-modulating effects. Many herbs have been screened for immuno-modulating activities in laboratories both within and beyond China. China has been applying an integrated approach to the treatment of AIDS. Immuno-enhancement herbs are used together with potent anti-viral drugs; 27%–67% improvements on the immunological status have been obtained.

Keywords: Chinese Medicine; AIDS; Herbal Therapy.

5.1 Introduction

AIDS is a global intractable pandemic. It has no vaccine, and cannot be cured at the present moment. However, the number of HIV-infected patients worldwide increases rapidly, particularly in developing countries. Treating these patients is a problem that remains to be solved. Since it has no cure, "to survive with HIV" is the optimal result that can be reached. The objective of treatment would be to elevate the quality of life, lower the AIDS morbidity and mortality, reduce the opportunistic infection, decrease the infectivity and prolong the survival period. To achieve this, every means should be used, including modern medicine (MM) and Chinese medicine (CM).

How can CM be used to treat HIV? What kind of approach and strategy would get the optimal outcome?

5.2 Reductional Analytical Approach

Reducing the research subject to a smaller entity to facilitate study of greater depth is a frequently used modern scientific approach. Focusing the level of study from organ to cell, molecule and gene, and subsequently reconstituting these studies, better results had been observed. Modern medicine has advanced from the uses of anti-HIV screening approaches in the early years to the recent understanding of the two vital enzymes for viral replication: the reverse transcriptase (RT, for transcription of DNA from RNA) and aspartyl protease (for proper virion assembly and maturation) and the subsequent discovering of their corresponding inhibitors. The breaking through of conventional monotherapy to combination therapy or "cocktail" (HAART) methods had attained higher efficacy of viral inhibition. During the 14th AIDS World Conference held in July 2002 in Barcelona, Spain, 924 various articles on HAART were published. This proved that this therapy can reduce the viral load to undetectable, alleviate symptoms, enhance immunity, lower morbidity and mortality and lower the opportunistic infection. The results are very promising; although it cannot annihilate HIV completely, but it proves to be a successful therapeutic approach.

One of the characteristics of CM is the holistic balanced approach. Reductional analytical approach is the modern scientific method, and CM has to use this approach in order to modernise itself.

In the past years, numerous Chinese herbs has been screened by various scientists. Chang and Yeung (1998) of the U.S. has screened 27 anti-infective herbs and found that 11 among them such as *Viola yedoensis*, *Prunella vulgaris*, *Lonicera japonica*, *Lithospermum erythrorhizon*,

Epimedium brevicornum, etc. have virus inhibitory effects. Luo *et al.* (1998) from China screened 700 Chinese herbs and found 141 species among them could inhibit HIV; herbs such as *Cortex morus alba*, *Croton tiglium*, *Rhaponticum uniflorum* have HIV inhibitory effects. However, due to constrained conditions, they have not conduct the enzyme inhibitory screening test. Watanabe (1989) of Japan has found that Minor Bupleurum Decoction (MBD) has anti-RT activity, and the inhibition rate reached 90%. He further investigated the components of MBD and found that *Scutellaria baicalensis* (baicalin and baicalein) was the effective herb of anti-RT effect. Xu *et al.* (1996) from Singapore has conducted the screening on protease inhibition (PI) of HIV and found that 19 among 75 herbs and their aqueous extracts such as *Anemarrhena aspheloides*, *Coptis chinensis*, *Epimedium brevicornum*, *Oldenlandia diffusa*, *Phellodendron chinense*, *Platycodon grandiflorum*, *Prunus mume*, *Punica granatum*, *Brucea javanica*, *Scutellaria baicalensis*, *Sophora japonica*, *Taraxacum mongolicum*, *Terminalia chebula*, *Belamcanda chinensis* and *Paeonia suffroticosa* have PI activity rates of over 70% at a concentration of 250 μg/ml using fluorogenic assay. However, among the extracts examined, if the concentration of 25 μg/ml of *Belamcanda chinensis*, *Paeonia suffroticosa*, *Phellodendron chinense* and *Terminaria chebula* was used, the PI inhibition rate were over 55%. Other herbs such as *Coptis chinensis*, *Versicolor coriolus* polysaccharide, *Lithospermum erythrorhizon*, *Salvia miltiorrhiza*, *Schizandra chinensis*, *Scutellaria baicalensis* (baicalin and baicalein) has anti-RT effect.

In the past 15 years, *Scutellaria baicalensis*, *Lithospermum erythrorhizon*, *Salvia miltiorrhiza* have been used for HIV-infected patients' treatments, but without the combined usage of RT inhibitors and PI in a planned way. However, they all showed improvement of immunity.

If the above-mentioned herbs were combined according to various species and dosages to formulate a noval compound recipe, such kind of simulation of HAART production would probably yield better results against HIV. When the target of study shifted from the virus to the enzyme of virus, it signifies progress in the methodology of the screening procedure. Of course, this is only the beginning, and many problems need further study.

5.3 Holistic Balanced Approach

CM holds that everything in the universe is constituted by Yin and Yang, and that they are the unity of opposites.

5.3.1 *Evil versus normal qi (spear versus shield)*

Yin-Yang dynamically balance results in healthy life, while an imbalance causes sickness. HIV is a pathogenic evil — the offensive "spear"; and the body resistance is normal qi — the defensive "shield". The evil and normal qi, as well as "spear" and "shield" are pairs of opposites — one gets sick when evil predominates, but recovers when normal qi predominates. MM stresses on the inhibition of HIV to weaken the offensive "spear", and stresses that the HIV is the only causative factor of AIDS. Inhibition of the HIV would either solve the problem of virus, and also support the body immunity. Some even holds that this approach will "kill two birds with one stone". Although it is important to inhibit the virus, the pathologic change it induced would not be wiped out by merely suppressing the etiologic factor — the pathogenesis involved would be improved by the change of immunity specifically. The strategy of MM is different from that of CM, but the aim for AIDS treatment is just the same. The therapeutic mechanism of anti-viral drug is "the inhibition of enzymes of HIV — the RT and protease — not the HIV-infected cells itself" (Levy, 2000).

In the foreword of his book *HIV and the Pathogenesis of AIDS*, Levy (2000) wrote "In recent years the most important trends is the shifting of the focal point to the immune system". However, during the Barcelona 14th World AIDS Conference, 924 clinical reports on HAART were presented, and only five articles were on immunotherapy. Therefore, the majority of clinical researcher is still concerned about the inhibition of HIV (Abstracts of XIV International Conference on AIDS).

5.3.2 *Immuno-enhancement should be the key*

There are two issues involved in the treatment for AIDS, namely, HIV and patient's immunological state. MM is different from CM. The former places emphasis on HIV, the latter on patient immunity. From the point of view of research thinking and methodology, MM has changed its focal point from virus to immunity, and this is an encouraging trend of AIDS research (Levy, 2000). It makes people consider the AIDS problem on a holistic approach. Because the offensive "spear" (HIV) attacks and destroys the chief defensive "shield" of the body (immunity), therefore one approach is to weaken the offensive "spear", and to strengthen the defensive "shield" is another.

This approach is particularly important to CM study in treating AIDS. CM is able to suppress HIV, but it is good in treating patients in a holistic manner by modulating the body immunity, through syndrome differentiation of HIV-infected patients, screening the effective herbs and confirming their efficacy.

In clinical practice, viral load reducing accompanied with immuno-enhancing (increase in CD_4^+ cells) is often encountered, but sometimes it is not so. Although HIV is inhibited to undetectable, but it has not been eliminated completely, the hypo-immunity also not recovered eventually. Therefore during treatment of an AIDS patient, both aspects of virus and patient should be considered concurrently.

Concentrating one's effort on seeking for new anti-viral agents is necessary, but one cannot have a one-track mind. If one sticks to inhibiting HIV, the more potent the anti-viral drug, the greater the damage on normal cells. The strategy of inhibiting virus as the sole means to solve the entire AIDS problem is not practical.

In defining anti-viral drugs, we usually stress on its ability in suppressing HIV, i.e. the result of viral load reduction is necessary. But the immune function elevation occurs while HIV is still present in the patient's body, and it still persistently destroys the immune competent cells. Those that can enhance the immunity of the HIV patient should be taken as auxiliary anti-viral agents. It is more appropriate to call them "anti-viral immuno-enhancers" so as to unify the two concepts of immunity and virus, bringing the immuno-enhancer into the category of anti-viral treatment.

At present, our strategy on AIDS research is: Welcome all the achievements obtained by MM and CM on anti-viral therapy respectively, and at the same time, give CM the role of full play in enhancing immunity. The focus should be seeking for specific immuno-enhancing herbs. Because the anti-viral agent study of MM has already reached a considerably high level, the present Chinese herbal study is not able to reach that level, and the study of minute virus with reductionism is not the strength of CM. The opinions of domestic scientists devoted to AIDS research gradually expressed unanimously that the immune aspect of CM should be the key focus. Because the holistic approach, syndrome differentiation and immune function strengthening are the merits of CM, we should develop these strong aspects and avoid the weakness so as to elevate the efficacy of CM.

In the past we have used recipes such as Glyke, Zhongyan I, Zhongyan II, Aitong, 21st Century Kangbao, and they all showed immunity improvement of 27%–67%, but without the data of viral load (Lu *et al.*, 2000). But later on, further studies were carried out, which showed that some efficacy was obtained. In 44 cases using Zhongyan II, five in 31 cases (16.31%) showed viral load reduction (> 0.5 log); two of them were undetectable; 44 cases were also tested for CD_4^+. The test results indicated that 11 of their CD_4^+ raised more than 50/mm^3; 12 of them changed less than 50/mm^3, which meant they remained stable (Guan *et al.*, 2003).

Recently, we used an effective anti-cancer agent, the Jinlong capsule (金龙胶囊) which consisted of fresh medicinal animals such as gecko, krait and viper in treating AIDS patients, and found that this capsule cannot significantly lower viral load. Only a small part of patients' viral load were lowered, but the elevation rate of CD_4^+ count reached 80% of patients, from 186.4 ± 110.92/mm^3 to 300.73 ± 164.57/mm^3, the mean elevation reached 114.33 ± 154.76/mm^3 (Lu, Wang and Li, 2003). This is a kind of non-specific immuno-enhancer — it elevates the immune function of both cancer patients and AIDS patients. Before the discovery of AIDS in 1981, CM was used to treat many hypo-immune asthenic syndromes such as chronic Xulao (虚劳) syndrome, cancer, congenital weak and repeated respiratory infection. They all were treated with similar immuno-enhancing agents like ginseng and deer antler (参茸) to strengthen the constitution and improve the disorder. If one uses the immuno-enhancing herbs and combine with viral inhibiting agents to formulate a potent compound anti-viral agent, it would certainly be beneficial for the treatment of HIV-infected patients.

For the whole world, if 1/10 of manpower, material and financial resource of AIDS research were put into the immunity research of AIDS patients constantly, a new undertaking on AIDS research would emerge. The key is to have a radical change on the strategic thought.

5.4 Integrative Complementary Approach

One could conduct a study on integrating CM and MM using a complementary approach that both inhibits the spear and strengthens the shield.

This includes using both CM and MM anti-viral drugs and immuno-enhancing agents of both types of medicines by taking advantage of the strengths of both medicines. In the acute stage when the viral load is high, HAART should be used, but when the viral load is reduced to undetectable, addition of the immuno-enhancing herbs of CM is preferred to consolidate the efficacy and prevent rebound. Or in the acute stage, when the viral load is high, administer HAART/immunotherapy = 9:1; while on the undetectable viral load, change the ratio to 3:7 or 1:9. The ratio could be adjusted to adapt to the changing condition of host and virus. The superiority of compound prescription should be emphasised. Good results have been displayed in inhibiting virus, and would play an even more important role in immuno-enhancement.

The above-mentioned three approaches have been summarised from the achievements of MM, as well as the practice of CM in treating AIDS. More research needs to be done in the future in this area.

References

Abstracts of XIV International Conference on AIDS (2002) Barcelona.

Chang, R.S. and Yeung, H.W. (1988) Inhibition of growth of human immunodeficiency virus *in vitro* by crude extracts of Chinese medicinal herbs. *Antiviral Res.* **9**, 163–175.

Guan, C.F., Wang, J., Xu, S.L., *et al.* (2003) Clinical and experimental study of Zhongyan II in treating AIDS. *Compil. 1st Natl. Integr. Chin. West Med. Treat. AIDS Acad. Symp.* **4**, 47–50.

Levy, J.A. (2000) *HIV and the Pathogenesis of AIDS*. Translated by Shao, Y.M., *et al.* Beijing Science Press.

Lu, W.B., Guan, C.F., *et al.* (2000) *Hope of AIDS Patients*. China Traditional Chinese Medicine Press, Beijing.

Lu, W.B., Wang, J. and Li, J.S. (2003) Preliminary report of Jinlong capsule in treating 20 HIV-infected patients. *Compil. 1st Natl. Integr. Chin. West. Med. Treat. AIDS Acad. Symp.* **4**, 56–59.

Luo, S.D., Fan, D.Q., Wang, H.Y., *et al.* (1998) *Chinese Herbal Study in Anti-HIV Activity*. Yunnan Science and Technology Press.

Watanabe, K. (1989) *Abstracts of V International Conference on AIDS*. Montreal.

Xu, H.X., Wan, M., Loh, B.N., *et al.* (1996) Screening of traditional medicine for their inhibitory activity against HIV-1 protease. *Phytother. Res.* **10**, 207–210.

Chapter 6

Anti-liver Fibrosis with Integrated Traditional Chinese and Western Medicine

Ping Liu, Cheng-hai Liu, Cheng Liu, Yi-yang Hu & Lie-ming Xu

Abstract

Liver cirrhosis is considered a pathological condition, which till today, is without an effective treatment. Chinese medicine, in the past three decades, has claimed successes in the treatment of this condition, through the use of single herbs or herbal formulae. Evaluation of the clinical effects has been based on simple observations, standard laboratory results and light or electron microscopy.

The herbs believed to be useful for liver cirrhosis are cordyceps, Fuzheng Huayu recipe, 861 recipe, Salvia root, etc. Molecular biology markers were used in the evaluation of these clinical trials.

It is suggested that in future research on liver cirrhosis, molecular biology can offer broader perspectives of evaluation. Multi-link and multi-level comprehensive anti-liver fibrosis mechanism of Chinese herbs may be worked out. More molecular details like TGF, mRNA expressions, factors affecting hepatic sinusoidal capillarisation and various intracellular single transductions, can be the targets of future research.

Keywords: Liver Cirrhosis; Chinese Medicine; Molecular Biology.

6.1 Introduction

Tissue fibrosis is a healing response to injuries featured with a process of extracellular matrix (ECM) over-production and deposition. Liver fibrosis is a common histological change of various chronic liver diseases through which the cirrhosis was developed. Nowadays, the prevention and reserving of liver fibrosis is an important therapeutic strategy because there is no special and effective therapy for primary diseases of liver fibrosis. Following cytokines being the popular approach to liver fibrosis, there has been fast development in the field of molecular biology and intracellular signaling for the study of liver fibrosis. Because it is hard to make a breakthrough for the therapeutics of liver fibrosis at present, emphasis should be put on fundamental research so as to seek a breakthrough from the highlighted mechanism of liver fibrosis and the invention of new drugs and therapy (Wang, 1997). However, TCM clinical and fundamental studies have shown significant superiority for treating liver fibrosis (Liu *et al.*, 1988). From the 1970s, the study of TCM in treating and preventing cirrhosis and liver fibrosis has been carried out and development has been achieved with the following ways: study from compound recipe, single drugs and effective ingredients; and study from naked eye observation, light microscopic pathological observation, electronic microscopic ultra structure changes and biochemical analysis. This paper outlines the progress in anti-liver fibrosis and looks into the future of this field.

6.2 Clinical Efficacy of TCM in Inhibiting Liver Fibrosis

In the past decade, anti-liver fibrosis study of TCM has been generally highly regarded and significant progress has been made with new drug put into clinical application.

6.2.1 *Peach kernel extract combined with cordyceps can improve the activity of interstitial collagenase and enhance the reversion of liver fibrosis*

In early 1980s, based on the theory of abdominal mass correlated to liver fibrosis, pains in both sides of the rib with varied position and occasional swelling of feet if evils settle in the liver is caused by extravagated blood stagnating internally (from Miraculous Pivot · Five Evil). Accumulation is due to evil *qi* settling resulted from *qi* deficiency. Focusing directly at two key factors: blood stasis and *qi* deficiency, and based on previous work, we applied cordyceps combining extract of peach kernel to inhibit liver fibrosis. The study was randomised, double blinded and controlled, with parameters as appearance under laparoscope, liver biopsy, collagen metabolism (collagenase activity of liver tissue, serum MAO activity, P-III-P, $\alpha 2$-macroglobin and urinary hydroxyproline content, etc.) and liver function, etc. The above-mentioned parameters reveal that peach kernel extract combined with cordyceps can enhance liver fibrosis reversion effectively, improve portal hypertension and regulate abnormal immune state. Experiments on rabbit schistosomiasis model suggest that anti-liver fibrosis effect of extract combining cordyceps is superior to any single drug among the two, and the main action mechanism is improvement of liver tissue collagenase activity and enhanced degradation of collagen in fibrotic liver (Liu *et al.*, 1988; Zhang *et al.*, 1988) (Figs. 6.1 and 6.2).

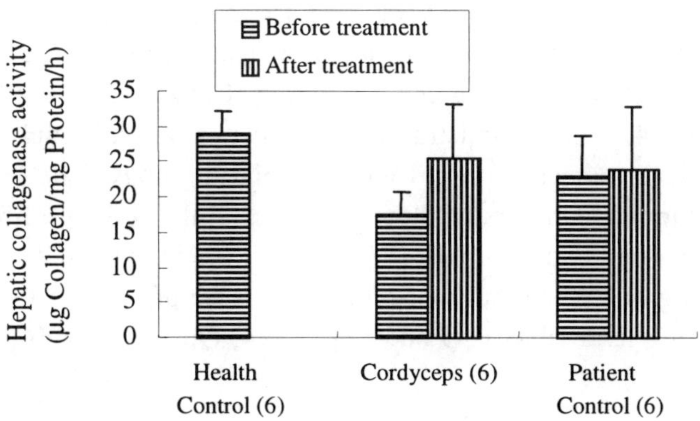

Figure 6.1. The effect of *Cordyceps Extract* on the collagenase activity in the schistosomiasis patients with hepatic fibrosis.

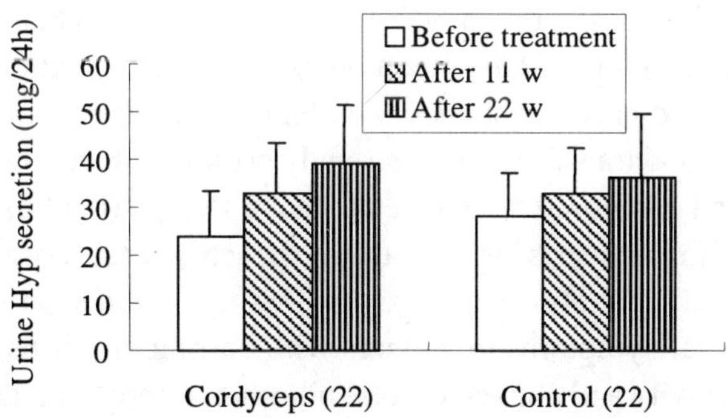

Figure 6.2. The effect of *Cordyceps Extract* on the urine Hyp secretion in the schistosomiasis patients with hepatic fibrosis.

Further studies on treating post-hepatitic cirrhosis with this recipe also showed good results — it can significantly increase patients' serum albumin content, decrease portal hypertension (widen portal vein diameter and decrease the size of swelling spleen), decrease serum MAO activity, decrease P-III-P and plasma Hyp content, improve abnormal immune state (improve cellular immunity, decrease serum IgG and IgA content) and clinical symptoms. Results from laparoscopic biopsy before and after treatment suggest that fibre accumulation decreases on liver surface, colour and luster changes from dark to ruddy, texture softens, falciform ligment oedema disappears, degree of omentum majus varices decreases; content of I and III type collagen, laminine (LM) fibronectine (FN) in hepatic septa decrease significantly compared to that of pre-treatment, HSC changes from activating state to quiescent state and hepatic sinusoidal capillarisation improves to a certain degree (Liu *et al.*, 1991; Xu *et al.*, 1993 and 1994). The administration of extract of peach kernel in patients with subsclera trabeculectomy by otorhinolaryngology. The Hospital of Shanghai Medical University shows that it can inhibit the proliferation of inflammatory cell and fibroblast (Wang *et al.*, 1993); there are also reports from Beijing and Shanghai that cordyceps is helpful in protecting liver and inhibiting liver fibrosis (Zhu *et al.*, 1994; Qiu *et al.*, 1997).

6.2.2 *Fuzheng Huayu Recipe can reverse liver fibrosis in chronic hepatitis B and has comprehensive effect on post-hepatitic cirrhosis*

In the late 1980s, based on pathomechanism of chronic hepatitis as dual deficiency of *qi* and Yin, static blood blocking vessels, pestilent dampness, heat lingering and previous studies, we established a therapeutic method of invigorating blood transforming stasis and boosting essence supplementing deficiency, and composed the Fuzheng Huayu Recipe (the Fuzheng Huayu Capsule (FZHY) consists of salvia root, peach kernel, cordyceps, etc.). Results from clinical observation reveal that this recipe can significantly improve clinical symptoms in patients with chronic hepatitis B, decrease serum ALT activity and content of total bilirubin, improve content of serum albumin and A/G ratio, significantly decrease abnormally increased serum liver fibrotic parameters as MAO activity, TIMP, P-III-P, IV type collagen,

HA and LM content (Liu *et al.*, 1996b). Laparoscope's examination reveals that fibrous bands decreases and inflammatory adhesion alleviates after treatment; liver biopsy reveals that liver cell degeneration and necrosis alleviates. Liver fibrosis reversion rate after treatment (lowers at least one stage after treatment) is 58.3%. After treatment, perisinosoidal I type collagen and LM decrease, IV type collagen increases (hepatic sinusoidal

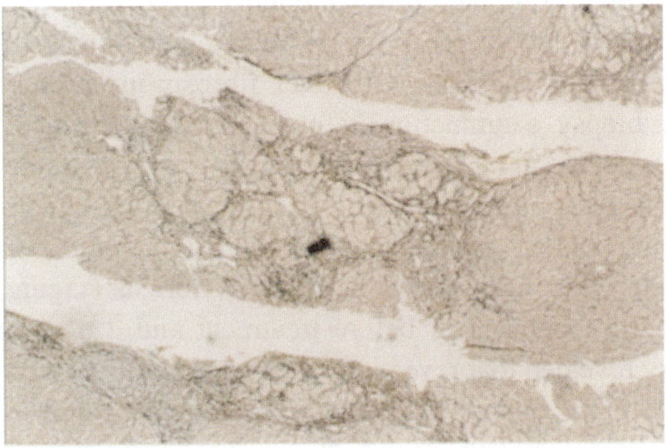

(a)

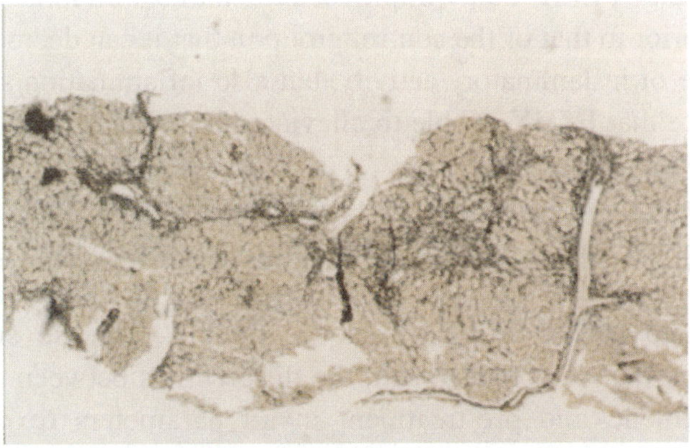

(b)

Figure 6.3. The effect of Fuzheng Huayu decoction on liver fibrosis in patient with chronic type B hepatitis: (a) before treatment and (b) after treatment.

structure recovered likely), I, III, IV type collagen expression decrease or disappear in most patients. All these suggest that this recipe is effective in treating chronic hepatitis B, especially in inhibiting liver fibrosis (Liu *et al.*, 1998c) (Fig. 6.3).

Furthermore, multi-center, randomised, double blinded and paralleled controlled trials were conducted on 216 patients with liver fibrosis in chronic hepatitis B (110 cases in trial group, 106 in control group, of which 99 cases in trial and 96 in the control group received histological diagnosis) in five centres receiving 24-week clinical treatment.

Results from 93 patients with liver fibrosis in chronic hepatitis B under liver biopsy examination before and after treatment reveal that liver fibrosis degree in FZHY decreases significantly with the mean value of liver fibrosis staging (S) in FZHY (50 cases) being 2.33 before treatment and 1.80 after FZHY treatment, while there is no improvement in the control group with the mean value of liver fibrosis staging (S) control group (43 cases) being 2.11 before treatment and 2.14 after treatment. Liver biopsy revealed that reversion rate (judged by liver fibrosis staging) is 52% in FZHY group and 23.3% in the control group, showing significant difference between the two groups. Histological examination showed that FZHY has obvious effect against liver fibrosis and is superior to that of Heluo Shugan capsule. Furthermore, liver histological examination also suggested that FZHY helps improve liver tissue inflammatory activity and is superior to that of the control group in that it can decrease not only mean value of inflammatory activity, but also inflammation score. These demonstrate that FZHY is able to alleviate inflammatory cell infiltration and or hepatic cell necrosis.

Parameters for liver fibrosis (HA, LM, P-III-P, IV-C) reveal that there is no significant difference in serum content of HA, LM, P-III-P, IV-C between the two groups before treatment. Each parameter in the FZHY group at 12- and 24-week treatments decrease significantly compared to that of pre-treatment, the differentials between 12- and 24-week treatment, and pre-treatment in all parameters (except LM at 24-week treatment) are significantly greater than that of the control group. The effectual is defined as two of four parameters of serum IV-C, HA, LN and P-III-P after treatment lowers equal to or more than 30% of baseline value compared to that of before treatment. According to this

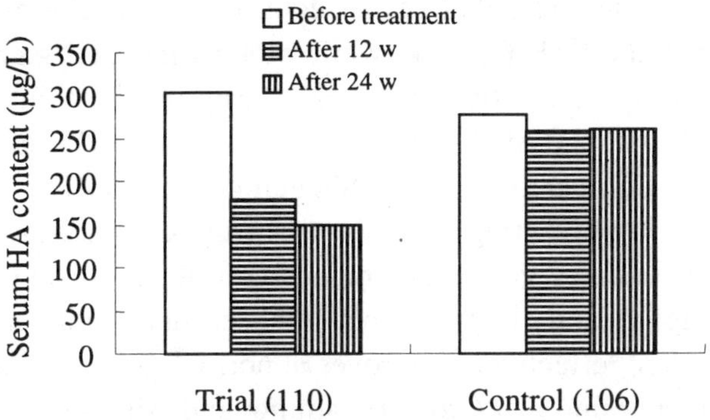

Figure 6.4. The effect of Fuzheng Huayu decoction on serum HA contents in patients with chronic type B hepatitis and liver fibrosis.

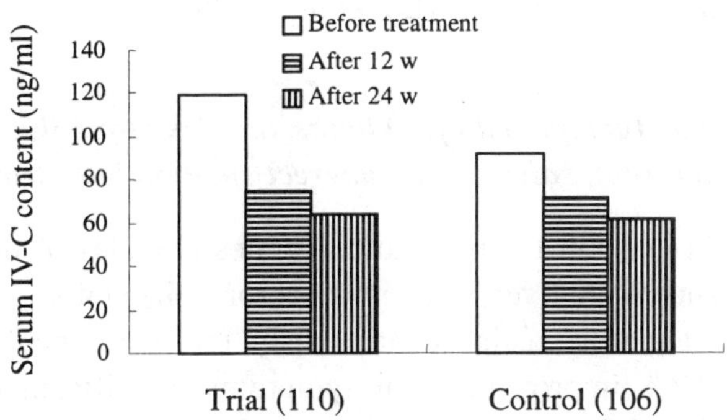

Figure 6.5. The effect of Fuzheng Huayu decoction on serum type IV collagen contents in patients with chronic type B hepatitis and liver fibrosis.

standard, the effectual rate in FZHY group is 72.7% and 27.4% in the control group. This indicates that Fuzheng Huayu Capsule is superior to Heluo Shugan Capsule in improving serum parameters for liver fibrosis in patients with liver fibrosis in chronic hepatitis B (Figs. 6.4 and 6.5).

There is no significant difference in serum TP, Alb, Glo, ALT, AST, GGT, ALP, T.bil and D.bil level between the two groups. The Alb, ALT, AST, GGT and ALP were significantly improved in both groups after treatment, indicating that both drugs have similar effects. The improvement in active GGT differential at 24-week treatment in the tester group is significantly greater than that of the control group. Albumin increases significantly in the FZHY group, while globins increase significantly in the control group. The effective rates of improvement in serum ALT activity are 72.7% and 59.4%, respectively in the FZHY group and the control group. Compared to Heluo Shugan capsule, FZHY is obviously more effective in preventing liver diseases from chroniclisation.

FZHY also shows good comprehensive effects on de-compensated cirrhosis: it significantly improves patients' serum albumin and decreases γ-globins content; effectively improves abnormal ratio of plasma ratio of branched chain amino acid/aromatic amino acid; significantly decreases patients' increased serum LM and HA content; raises the number of CD^{+3}, CD^{+4}, ratio of CD^{+4}/CD^{+8}, NK cell activity and complement C3 content; decreases serum IgG and IgM content; and it regulates abnormal changes of endocrine hormone (Liu *et al.*, 1996c).

6.2.3 *861 recipe (comprised of 10 herbs such as mongolian milkvetch root, salvia root, suberect spatholobus stem, etc.)*

The Beijing Friendship Hospital administrates granules of this recipe in treating patients with liver fibrosis in chronic hepatitis B. Forty-nine patients who took the recipe continuously for more than half a year experienced 67% improvement in symptoms, significant decrease in serum P-III-P and LM content compared to that of pre-treatment and 73% recovery rate in ALT activity. Among them, 33% of the patients experienced portal vein diameter decrease and 52% retraction rate of swelling spleen. Biopsy from 12 patients with six-month administration before and after treatment reveals that this recipe can alleviate the degree of liver fibrosis synchronising to the improvement in liver tissue inflammation (Zhao *et al.*, 1997). *In vivo* and *in vitro* experiments also indicate that this recipe can inhibit transcription of collagen gene (Wang, 1996).

6.2.4 *Salvia root and its effective ingredients*

In the early 1950s, there were reports on salvia decoction in treating splenomegaly in terminal schistosomiasis (Wu *et al.*, 1958). In recent years, salvia root is widely used in treating chronic hepatitis B and early stage post-hepatitic cirrhosis, because its anti-liver fibrosis effect might be its key link in treating these diseases (Liu *et al.*, 1998a). Salvia root injection is used clinically in treating chronic hepatitis B, and pre- and post-treatment liver biopsy reveal that it can effectively improve pathological changes in liver fibrosis (Yu *et al.*, 1994). Dynamic ultrasound Doppler examination of patients with post-hepatitic cirrhosis receiving salvia root injection reveal that it can effectively increase portal vein blood flow (Li *et al.*, 1996). During the period of the Ninth Five Year Plan, we assumed the national project of tackling key problem in science and technology — research on salvianolic acid B in inhibiting liver fibrosis in chronic hepatitis B. A randomised, double blinded controlled and double dummy method was used in this study. Patients with chronic hepatitis B took SA-B and received intramuscular injection of IFN-γ respectively, and at same time, patients were given corresponding imitated blank preparation. There were 30 patients in both the observation and the control groups, and all patients went through six months of treatment. Therapeutic effect was judged mainly by histological examination (all the patients had complete liver biopsy data pre- and post-treatment and were determined blindly by three pathologists) and combined with symptoms and signs before, during and after treatment, virology and liver function examination, serological parameters for liver fibrosis (HA, LM, C-IV, P-III-P), B ultrasound examination of liver and routine safety examination during administration. Results reveal that: (1) liver fibrosis reversion rate in SA-B group is 36.67% (11/30) and inflammation improvement rate is 40.0% (12/30), while that of the γ-IFN group is 30.0% (9/30) and 36.67% (11/30) respectively; (2) HA and C-IV content decrease significantly after SA-B treatment. The above-mentioned decreases in serological parameters for liver fibrosis indicate that improvement in the treatment group is significantly superior to that of the control group; (3) there is no significant difference between the two groups in improvement in liver function, symptoms and signs; (4) the score of B ultrasound improvement in the SA-B group is superior to the IFN-γ group; (5) ALT, AST activity and total bilirubin in patients with liver fibrosis reversion in SA-B group before treatment are significantly lower than that of liver fibrosis aggravating patients; (6) IFN-γ has side effects to a certain degree (fever and transient decrease of leukocyte with incidence rates of 50% and 3.23%, respectively), while SA-B has no obvious side effect; and (7) serum parameters for liver fibrosis correlate positively to the degree of liver fibrosis and inflammation in general. Each parameter increases to a certain degree accompanying aggravation of liver fibrosis and inflammation. This initial experiment indicates that SA-B can effectively reverse liver fibrosis in chronic hepatitis B (histological reversion rate is 36.67%); SA-B's effect on serum HA content is superior to that of IFN-γ; and liver fibrosis in

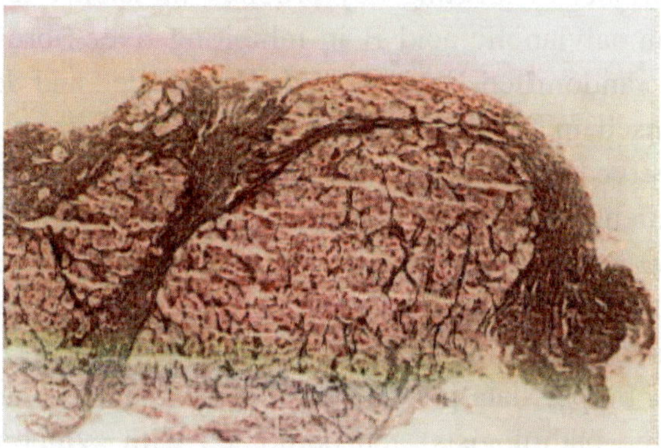

(a)

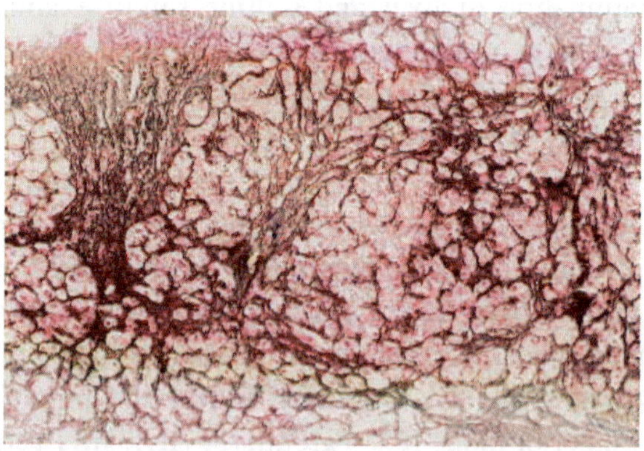

(b)

Figure 6.6. The effect of SA-B liver fibrosis in patient with chronic type B hepatitis: (a) before treatment and (b) after treatment.

chronic hepatitis B is more suitable for SA-B therapy (Liu *et al.*, 1998d) (Fig. 6.6).

6.3 Multi-Link and Multi-Level Comprehensive Anti-Liver Fibrosis Mechanism of Chinese Herbs

The formation and development of liver fibrosis is a rather complicated process, so it is beneficial for us to bring to light the comprehensive advantage of compound recipe of Chinese herbs in inhibiting liver fibrosis from multi-link or multi-level — Chinese herbs are characterised by multi-ingredients.

6.3.1 *Inhibiting fibre proliferating stimulating factor, HSC proliferation, TGFβ1 and collagen mRNA expression*

Pharmacodynamics experiment result indicate that FZHY can not only inhibit liver fibrosis formation induced by CCl_4, but can also enhance reversion of cirrhosis in rats induced by CCl_4 and dimethylnitrosamine (DMN) (Liu *et al.*, 1997b and c). Lipid peroxidation product MDA is the fibre proliferation stimulating factor which can significantly enhance HSC proliferation, type I collagen mRNA expression and production of collagen. MDA content in liver tissue in rats with chronic liver injury induced by CCl_4 increases significantly and correlates positively to Hyp content in liver tissue. The recipe can significantly decrease MDA content in liver tissue, indicating that anti-liver fibrosis effect of FZHY is correlated to anti-lipid peroxidation. *In vitro* experiments on cells isolated from chronic liver injury model after administration and cells that are treated with drug serum suggest that FZHY can significantly inhibit activation and proliferation of HSC, inhibit PDGF-BB stimulated HSC proliferation, inhibit TGF-β1 mRNA and its protein expression of HSC, and inhibit collagen mRNA and protein expression. Further recipe-splitting research reveal that stasis transforming drugs in the recipe has the strongest effect on inhibiting HSC proliferation and activation, right supporting drugs have the best effect on inhibiting type I collagen mRNA and protein expression and cordyceps have the most obvious effect on decreasing TGF-β1 mRNA

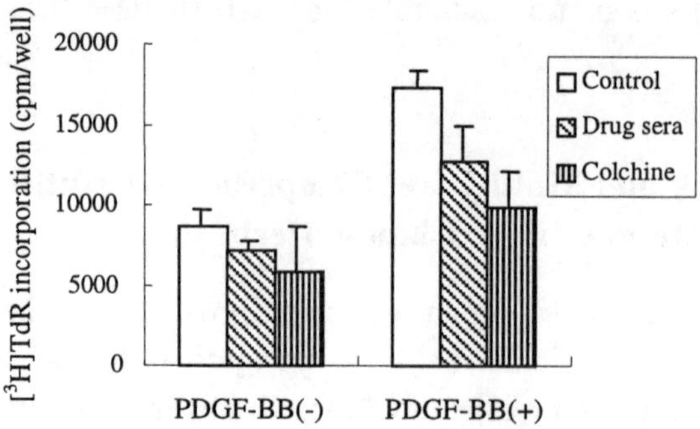

Figure 6.7. The effect of drug sera containing Fuzheng Huayu decoction on PDGF-bb stimulated rat HSC proliferation.

and protein expression. Experiments on immune injury liver fibrosis in rats induced by bovine albumin indicate that inhibiting the expression of hepatic TGF-β1 and its receptor is the major action mechanism of cordyceps and its effective ingredient-cordyceps polysaccharide against liver fibrosis. The recipe can also inhibit the proliferation of NIH/3T3 or fibroblast, decrease intra or extra collagen generation rate and mRNA expression of I, III, IV type collagen and type I collagen mRNA expression. Compound recipe can enhance reversion of liver fibrosis through regulating interstitial collagenase activity (Hu *et al.*, 1997; Liu *et al.*, 1996a, 1997a, 1998a and d, 1999 and 2002c) (Fig. 6.7).

Normal rat's Küpffer cell culture medium (NKcM) has no effect on HSC proliferation, while from the conditioned Küpffer cell medium from acute CCl_4 injured rats (IKcM) can significantly enhance HSC proliferation and type I collagen secretion, in a time- and dose-dependent manner. FZHY drug serum added to a conditioned Küpffer cell medium (Y-KcM) can significantly inhibit IKcM stimulated HSC proliferation and collagen secretion. Content of PDGF, TGFβ1 and vascular endothelial growth factor (VEGF) in IKcM increases significantly than that in NKCM and is predominantly the increase of active type TGFβ1. Recipe of Chinese herbs can markedly inhibit secretion of PDGF and TGFβ in Y-KcM (predominantly inhibit active type TGFβ) and also has some effect on inhibiting secretion of VEGF. *In vitro* subculturing HSC secretes more

TGFβ1 and VEGF than primary HSC, and Chinese herbs also shows the same significant inhibiting effect. Activated HSC conditioned medium can significantly enhance primary HSC proliferation and type I collagen secretion, while Chinese herbs added to an activated HSC conditioned medium can significantly inhibit HSC proliferation and type I collagen secretion. This indicates that compound recipe of Chinese herbs can inhibit the formation and development of liver fibrosis through inhibiting KC's paracrine and HSC's autocrine (Jiang *et al.*, 2000; Liu *et al.*, 2001a and b) (Figs. 6.8–6.10).

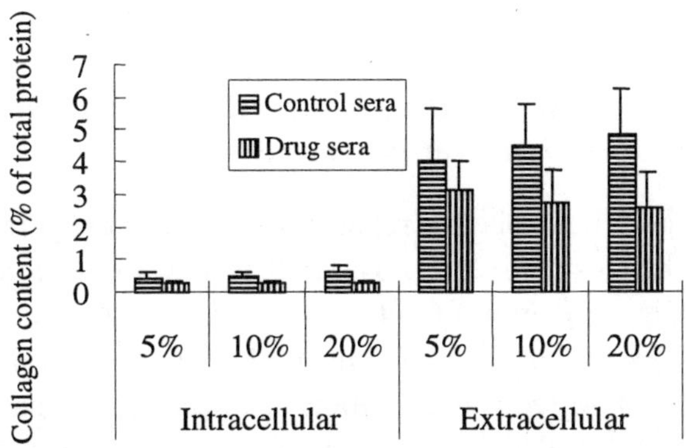

Figure 6.8. The effect of drug sera containing Fuzheng Huayu decoction on the collagen production in rat HSC. HSC was incubated with 5%–20% the drug sera for 48 h.

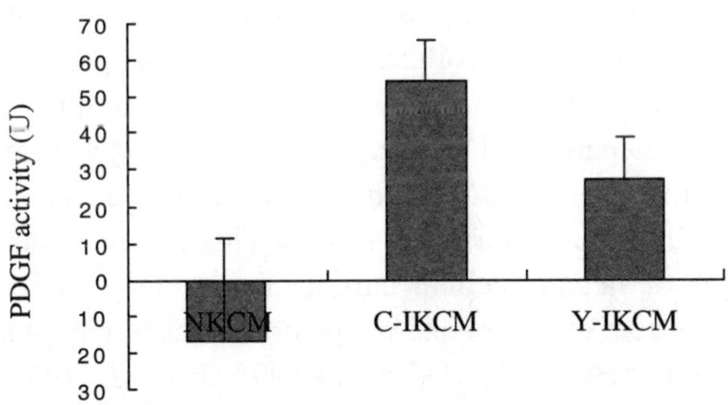

Figure 6.9. The effect of drug sera containing Fuzheng Huayu decoction on the PDGF secretion in Küpffer cells from acute injured liver by CCl_4.

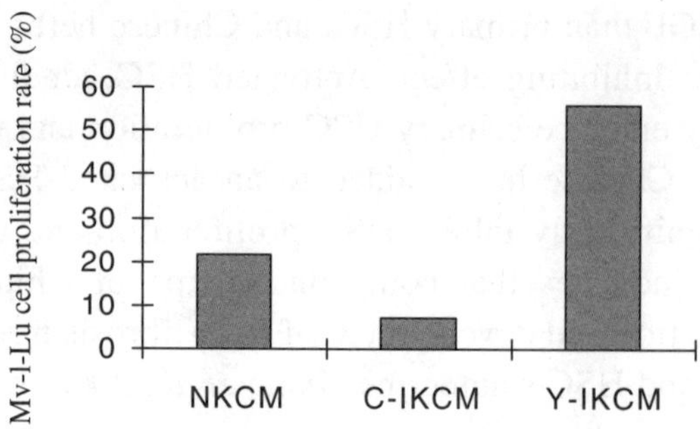

Figure 6.10. The effect of drug sera containing Fuzheng Hueyu decoction on the TGF-β activity in Küpffer cells from acute injured liver by CCl_4.

6.3.2 *Anti-liver injury, protecting hepatocyte and improving the recovery of chronic liver injured cells*

Hepatocyte injury, necrosis and regeneration have a close relationship to pathological changes of liver fibrosis in that liver injury initiating factor for liver fibrosis, activation of cell in sinusoidal wall in necrotic region is not only an important factor for liver fibrosis, but also an inexorable phenomenon for liver cell regeneration. These indicate that hepatic cell directly participate in the process of liver fibrosis in chronic liver injury. The FZHY recipe can not only inhibit lipid peroxidation and prevent structural and functional destruction of hepatic cell membrane caused by lipid peroxidation, but it can also improve Ca^{++}-ATPase activity and maintain Ca^{++} homeostasis in plasma and protect hepatic cell. The effect of FZHY on hepatic cell proliferation depends on pathophysiological state of cell because drug serum can enhance DNA synthesis of primary cell of rat and hepatic cell in acute liver injury. It has an inhibiting effect on already lowered DNA synthesis in CCl_4-induced chronic liver injury and DMN-induced cirrhosis in rats. This indicates that biological characteristics of hepatic cell in chronic liver injury has changed and the regulating effect of compound recipe correlates to pathophysiological state of liver cell (Hu *et al.*, 1997b and 1998; Ji *et al.*, 1997; Liu *et al.*, 1998b and 2001c).

The quantity of intra- and extra-cellular collagen of normal hepatic cell is 0.3% of its total albumen respectively, but the quantity of *in vitro*

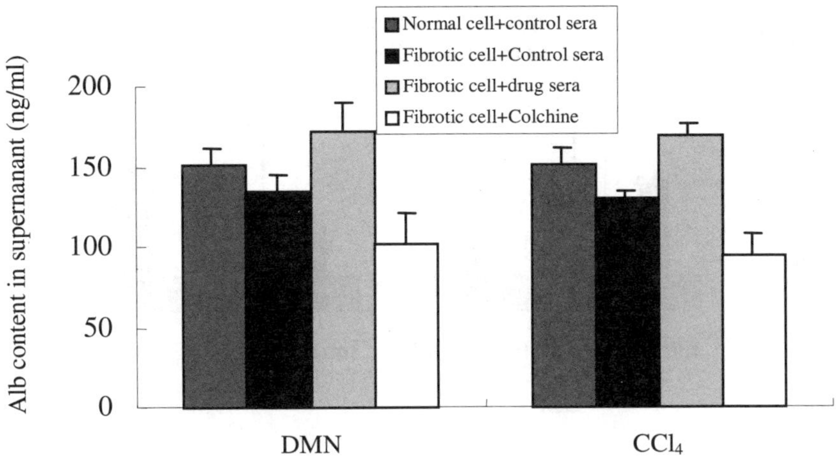

Figure 6.11. The effect of drug sera containing Fuzheng Hueyu decoction on the Alb secretion in hepatocytes from fibrotic liver.

acute injured hepatic cell increases by 40%, the quantity of intracellular collagen of chronic injured hepatic cell increases 1.5 times, the quantity of extracellular collagen of chronic injured hepatic cell increases 3.5 times, while the production of albumin decreases 14%. This indicates that albumin-producing function of chronic injured hepatic cell decreases while collagen (ECM, etc.)-producing function increases significantly (Fig. 6.11).

In vitro experiments reveal that the albumin-producing function of hepatic cells isolated from the liver of rats with chronic CCl_4 injury and DMN-induced cirrhosis decreases significantly. Drug serum of the compound recipe can promote its recovery to normal level and inhibit abnormal increased production of intra- and extra-cellular collagen. *In vivo* experiments also reveal that compound recipe is of the same action characteristics in that Alb mRNA expression (Northern blot) in the liver of DMN-induced cirrhosis decreases significantly and Alb mRNA expression increases significantly after treatment with the compound recipe. So we can conclude that FZHY can promote the functional recovery of chronic injured hepatic cell (Fig. 6.12).

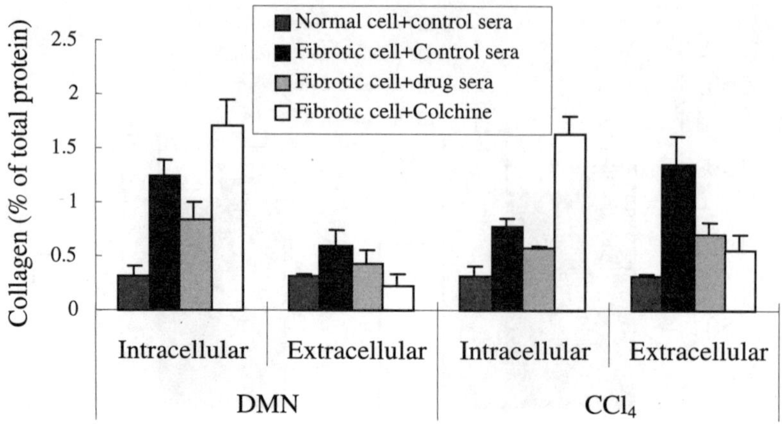

Figure 6.12. The effect of drug sera containing Fuzheng Hueyu decoction on the collagen synthesis in hepatocytes from fibrotic liver.

6.3.3 *Action of compound recipe of Chinese herbs on inhibiting hepatic sinusoidal capillarisation*

There is no definite conclusion on whether hepatic capillarisation can be reversed. During the process of DMN-induced liver fibrosis, loss of fenestra is obviously earlier than hepatic cell injury and formation of fibre septa and basement membrane under hepatic endothelium. After withdrawal of DMN, hepatic sinusoidal capillarisation alleviates spontaneously and its reversion is earlier than that of liver fibrosis. FZHY can significantly improve twisting and occlusion of hepatic sinus in rats with DMN-induced liver fibrosis and alleviate loss of fenestra in hepatic sinusoidal endothelium and formation of basement membrane under endothelium. The expression of VIII factor related antigen, LM, IV type collagen and α-smooth muscle actin (α-SMA) in hepatic sinusoidal wall decreases significantly — this indicates that FZHY can promote reversion of hepatic sinusoidal capillarisation in rats with liver fibrosis. The multilevel pharmacological effect of the compound recipe is the advantage of compound recipe in inhibiting liver fibrosis through regulating cellular function and its related functional gene (Lu *et al.*, 2000, 2002 and 2003).

6.3.4 *Action mechanism of salvianolic acid B(SA-B) (effective anti-liver fibrosis ingredient of salvia) on TGF-β1 intracellular signal transduction*

TGFβ1 can promote collagen secretion of quiescent, interim activated and complete activated HSC with promoting rates of 128.6%, 207.3% and 188.2%, respectively. Interim activated HSC is most sensitive to TGF-β1's collagen secretion enhancing effect; 0.1 μmol/L~1 μmol/L SA-B has no effect on cell form, but concentration can dependently inhibit HSC proliferation with intracellular [^{3}H] thymine impulsion as that of control group's 76.0%, 60.1% and 47.8%, respectively; 1 μmol/L~10 μmol/L SA-B can significantly inhibit TGFβ1 stimulated HSC collagen secretion (as that of control group's 68.6% and 56.1%), inhibit α-SMA and plasmin activator inhibitor −1 (PAI-1) protein expression, and downregulate type I collagen gene expression; 0.1 μmol/L~1 μmol/L SA-B can inhibit Smad2/3 protein expression at a varying degree and significantly inhibit intracellular phosphorylation and nuclear transposition of Smad2 protein. This suggests that the main action mechanism of SA-B in inhibiting liver fibrosis is to inhibit intracellular signal transduction of TGFβ1 in HSC and antagonise HSC activation promoting effect of TGFβ1 (Liu *et al.*, 2002a and b) (Fig. 6.13).

Based on overall advantage of TCM in inhibiting liver fibrosis and grasping complicated pathological changes in liver fibrosis, we should

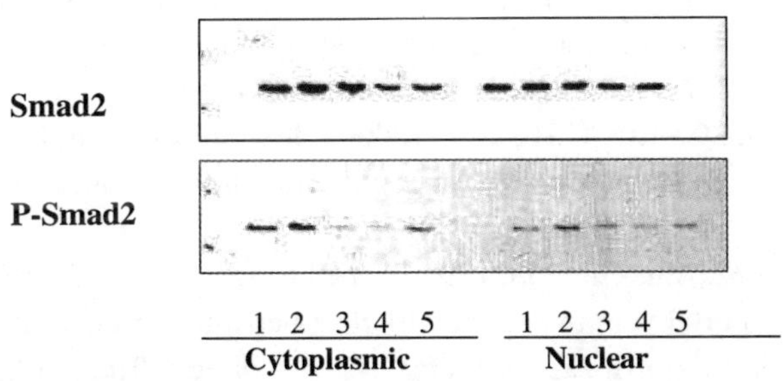

Figure 6.13. The effect of SA-B on TGF-β1 stimulated levels of Smad2 expression, phosphorylation and nucleus translocation in HSC. Western blot, lanes 1–5 stand for: Normal; Control (100 pM TGF-β1); 0.1 μM SA-B treated; 1 μM SA-B treated; and 10 μM SA-B treated.

focus on key pathological links of liver fibrosis which modern biological medicine is directed, and adopt such a research method of blocking or enhancing expression of some single ingredients. In doing so, we can promote the advantage of TCM in regulating functional gene to study the scientific theoretical basis of TCM in reversing liver fibrosis. Only in this way can we find a new liver fibrosis reversing ingredient or a new action of a known ingredient, disclose action mechanism of TCM in regulating functional gene (liver fibrosis related cytokine and extracellular matrix) and lay a sound theoretical foundation for TCM in reversing liver fibrosis and even early stage cirrhosis. This kind of approach may result in breakthroughs for TCM in treating serious diseases.

References

Hu, Y.Y., Liu, C., Liu, P., *et al.* (1997a) Anti-liver fibrosis of Fuzheng Huayu: recipe on CCl_4 induced liver fibrosis in rats and its relationship with anti-lipid peroxidation. *New J. Gastroenterol.* **5**(8), 5–6.

Hu, Y.Y., Liu, P., Liu, C., *et al.* (1997b) Dynamic changes of superoxide dismutase (SOD) and malonaldehyde in acute liver injury induced by CCl_4 intoxication and effect of Fuzheng Huayu decoction on them. *J. Integr. Tradit. West. Med. Liver Dis.* **7**(2), 87–89.

Hu, Y.Y., Liu, P., Liu, C., *et al.* (1998) Effect of Fuzheng Huayu recipe on Alb mRNA expression in liver in rats with DMN induced liver fibrosis. *New J. Gastroenterol.* **5**(8), 512–514.

Ji, G., Liu, P., Liu, C., *et al.* (1997) Effect of sera from the rat treated with Fuzheng Huayu decoction on rat hepatocyte proliferation and collagen synthesis *in vitro*. *Chin. J. Exp. Tradit. Med. Form.* **3**(3), 20–23.

Jiang, C.M., Liu, C., Liu, C.H., *et al.* (2000) Effect of Fuzheng Huayu decoction on function of Küppfer cell from acute injured liver induced by CCl_4. *Chin. J. Integr. Tradit. West. Med.* **10**(5), 26–28.

Li, C., Xue, H.M., Lu, G., *et al.* (1996) The changes of blood stream volume at the hepatic portal vein in patient with post-hepatitic cirrhosis and the effect of radix salvia miltiorrhizae on them. *Chin. J. Integr. Tradit. West. Med.* **6**(4), 3–6.

Liu, C., Jiang, C.M., Liu, P., *et al.* (2001a) Intervention of Fuzheng Huayu decoction on autocrine activation of hepatic stellate cells. *Chin. J. Hepatol.* **9**(5), 282–284.

Liu, C., Jiang, C.M., Liu, P., *et al.* (2001b) Effect of Fuzheng Huayu decoction on paracrine activation of hepatic stellate cells. *Chin. J. Dig.* **21**(6), 367–369.

Liu, C., Liu, P., Xu, L.M., *et al.* (1991) Observation of extractum semen persicae and cordyceps hyphae in treating post-hepatitic cirrhosis. *J. Tradit. Chin. Med.* **32**(7), 404–407.

Liu, C.H., Liu, C., Liu, P., *et al.* (1996a) Effect of sera containing Fuzheng Huayu decoction on Ito cell proliferation and collagen synthesis in rats. *Chin. J. Exp. Tradit. Med. Form.* **2**(2), 16–19.

Liu, C.H., Liu, C., Liu, P., *et al.* (1997a) Seropharmological effects of Fuzheng Huayu decoction on rat Ito cell morphology and function in culture. *China Natl. J. New Gastroenterol.* **3**(4), 263–265.

Liu, C.H., Liu, P., Hu, Y.Y., *et al.* (2002a) Effect of salvianolic acid B on TGF-β1 stimulated hepatic stellate cell activation and its intracellular signaling. *Natl. J. Chin. Med.* **82**(18), 1267–1272.

Liu, C.H., Wang, X.L., Tang, Y.Z., *et al.* (2001c) Herb compatible action of Fuzheng Huayu 319 recipe of albumin production in hepatocyte. *Chin. J. Basic Med. Tradit. Chin. Med.* **7**(4), 36–38.

Liu, P., Fang, B.W., Liu, C., *et al.* (1998a) The role of transforming growth factor-β1 and its effect on immunologically induced liver fibrogenesis and cordyceps polysaccharide on them. *Chin. J. Hepatol.* **6**(4), 232–234.

Liu, P., Hu, Y.Y., Liu, C.H., *et al.* (1997b) Anti-liver fibrosis effect of Fuzheng Huayu: recipe on DMN induced liver fibrosis and its effect on fat storing cell. *Chin. J. Tech. Tradit. Chin. Med.* **4**(2), 99–101.

Liu, P., Hu, Y.Y., Xu, L.M., *et al.* (1997c) Studying anti-fibrosis of liver with Fuzheng Huayu 319 recipe. *Chin. J. Exp. Tradit. Med. Form.* **3**(4), 20–24.

Liu, P., Ji, G., Hong, J.H., *et al.* (1998b) Changes of albumin and collagen formation of hepatic cell isolated from CCl_4 induced liver fibrosis and effect of sera of herb on it. *Chin. J. Hepatol.* **6**, 50–51.

Liu, P., Liu, C., Chen, G.C., *et al.* (1996b) Effect of Fuzheng Huayu 319 recipe on serological parameters of fibrosis in treating chronic hepatitis B. *Chin. J. Integr. Tradit. West. Med.* **16**(10), 588–592.

Liu, P., Liu, C., Xu. L.M., *et al.* (1998c) Effects of Fuzheng Huayu 319 recipe on liver fibrosis in chronic hepatitis B. *West. J. Gastroenterol.* **4**(4), 348–353.

Liu, P, Liu, C.H., Liu, C. and Xu, L.M. (1998d) Serum pharmacological study about effects of Fuzheng Huayu recipe on hepatic stellate cell proliferation and collagen synthesis in rats. *Chin. J. Integr. Med.* **4**(3), 118–122.

Liu, P., Liu, C.H., Wang, H.N., *et al.* (2002b) Effect of salvianolic acid B on collagen production and mitogen activated protein kinase activity in rat hepatic stellate cells. *Acta Pharmacol. Sin.* **23**(8), 7733–7738.

Liu, P., Liu, C.H., Yi, Y., *et al.* (1996c) Effect of Fuzheng Huayu 319 recipe in treating post-hepatitic cirrhosis. *Chin. J. Integr. Tradit. West. Med.* **16**(8), 459–462.

Liu, P., Wang, X.L., Liu, C.H., *et al.* (1999) Study on function of anti-pathogenic ability — supplementing and stagnation-dispersing compatibility influential to hepatic stellate cell activation, collagen formation and albumin formation of hepatocyte. *Acta Shanghai Univ. Tradit. Chin. Med.* **13**(3), 46–50.

Liu, P., Wu, D.Z., Liu, C.H., *et al.* (2002c) Mechanism study on combination of Chinese herbal formulae to support anti-pathogenic ability and dissipate blood stasis in promoting reversion of liver fibrosis in CCl_4 rats. *Acta Shanghai Univ. Tradit. Chin. Med.* **16**(1), 37–41.

Liu, P., Zhang, L.B., Liu, C., *et al.* (1988) Study on extractum semen persicae and cordyceps hyphae for resistance of hepatocirrhosis. II. Study on its effect on collagen metabolism in patients with schistosomiasis. *Acta Shanghai Univ. Tradit. Chin. Med.* **2**(1), 22–29.

Lu, X., Liu, P., *et al.* (2003) Effect of Fuzheng Huayu 319 recipe on hepatic sinusoidal capillarisation in rat induced with DMN. *J. Tradit. Chin. Med.* **44**(2), 136–139.

Lu, X., Liu, P., Liu, C.H., *et al.* (2002) Role of hepatic sinusoidal endothelium injury in hepatic fibrogenesis induced by dimethyltrosamine. *Chin. J. Gastroenterol.* **10**(6), 441–444.

Lu, X., Xu, G.F., Chen, W.H., *et al.* (2000) Dynamic changes of hepatic sinusoidal capillarisation. *West. J. Gastroenterol.* **8**(12), 1415–1416.

Qiu, D.K., Li, H., Zeng, M.D., *et al.* (1997) Effect of cordyceps polysacchride liposome on collagenase mRNA in rats with liver fibrosis. *New J. Gastroenterol.* **5**(7), 417–418.

Wang, B. (1996) Effect of herbal CPD 861 on collagen mRNA in liver of experimental fibrosis in rats. *Chin. J. Hepatol.* **4**(4), 214–216.

Wang, B. (1997) Generation and degeneration of extracellular matrix in hepatofibrosis. *Chin. J. Hepatol.* **5**(2), 65.

Wang, S.P., Fang, J., Ji, C.W., *et al.* (1993) Experimental study of extractum semen persicae in inhibiting fibroblastic proliferation after trabeculectomy. *Acta Shanghai Med. Univ.* **20**(1), 35–38.

Wu, Y.S., Yang, C.H., Jian, J.F., *et al.* (1958) Preliminary study of the effect of salvia on terminal stage schistosomiasis cirrhosis with splemomegaly. *Chin. J. Med.* **6**, 542–545.

Xu, L.M., Liu, P., Liu, C., *et al.* (1993) Effect of extractum semen persiae and cordyceps hyphae on appearance of ultra-microstructure and fat storing cell of liver in post-hepatitic cirrhosis patients. *J. Hepatol.* **1**, 9–11.

Xu, L.M., Liu, P., Liu, C. *et al.* (1994) Pathological and immunohistochemical study of extractum semen persiae and cordyceps hyphae in treating post-hepatitic cirrhosis. *J. Tradit. Chin. Med.* **35**, 737–739.

Yu, YX., Yang, H.Q., Zhu, L.Z., *et al.* (1994) Clinical observation on treating cirrhosis with heavy dose of radix salviae miltiorrhizae. *Shanghai J. Tradit. Chin. Med.* 2, 8–10.

Zhang. L.B., Liu, C., Xu, L.M., *et al.* (1988) Study on extractum semen persicae and cordyceps hyphae for resistance of hepatocirrhosis. III. Morphological study on 12 cases fibrosis. *Acta Shanghai Univ. Tradit. Chin. Med.* **2**(2), 22–23.

Zhao, H.T., Wang, T.L., *et al.* (1997) Istopathological evaluation of the therapeutic effect of herbal CPD 861 on liver fibrosis. *Chin. J. Hepatol.* **5**(2), 77–78.

Zhu, J.X., Wang, B.E. and Wang, T.L. (1994) Study on the therapeutic effect of cordyceps mycelium on experimental hepatic fibrosis of rat. *Chin. J. Dig.* **14**(6), 333–335.

Chapter 7

Advances in the Treatment of Lung Cancer by Traditional Chinese Medicine

Jia-xiang Liu

Abstract

The article reviews the advances in the fields of aetiology and pathology, treatment based on syndrome differentiation, therapeutic principles, specific prescriptions, new drugs and agents, and therapy with a combination of TCM and Western medicine in the past 20 years. It is believed that therapy based on comprehensive consideration with multi-targets is one of the keys to treating lung cancer with TCM in China. The treatment of lung cancer with TCM is mainly characterised by high stable rate of focus, long survival period, good quality of life, and potentially less chance for relapse and metastasis. The author feels that it is important to study survival period and quality of life, the combination therapy and assessment standard of therapeutic effect that is suitable for the situation in China, try to further unite and improve the types of syndrome, and study the nature of the types of syndrome for the purpose of improving the therapeutic effect of treating lung cancer.

Keywords: Lung Cancer, Therapy with TCM; Therapy of Combination of TCM and Western Medicine.

7.1 Introduction

Although prognosis of early lung cancer treated by surgery is effective, 86% of lung cancer patients are at the advanced stage when diagnosed. As only a small percentage of patients are operable, most are commonly treated by radiotherapy and chemotherapy. Although some patients get short-term therapeutic effect, the remission time, side effects and survival period are not satisfactory. Hence, prognosis of lung cancer is very poor. About 80% of patients die within one year after being diagnosed. Median survival period is about 6 months. Total survival rate of 5 years is only 5%–10% (Liu, 1996), and the therapeutic effect is not satisfactory. Its death rate is the highest for all malignant tumours and it was the main cause of death in the last 20 years (Li *et al.*, 1997). Hence, early diagnosis and early treatment were emphasised in recent years. It is recommended that middle and advanced stage patients should be treated by combined therapy with several subjects so as to improve therapeutic effect, prolong survival period and increase quality of life. The study of therapy of lung cancer with TCM or combination of TCM and Western medicine is very important. In recent years, there is a trend to differentiate syndrome and disease, strengthen the body resistance and eliminate the pathogenic factor to treat lung cancer with TCM or combination of TCM and Western medicine. These therapies have demonstrated positive results in the remission of symptoms, improving living quality, stabilising focus, prolonging survival period and increasing survival rate. Combined with surgery, radiotherapy and chemotherapy, TCM can also decrease side effects and increase clinical therapeutic effects. Some progress has been made in the fields of mechanism of the action of therapeutic effect with clinical trials and animal experiments through modern scientific methods, showing the importance of TCM in preventing and treating lung cancer.

7.2 Aetiology and Pathogenesis

The aetiological factor of lung cancer has not been clarified completely. Some scholars study pathogenesis based on the relative recordation of documents in all dynasties, and the genesis process and clinical situation. These studies mainly include three aspects:

(a) Based on the theory of deficiency of vital-qi, the imbalance between Yin and Yang of the viscera, and the deficiency of vital-qi are the internal causes of illnesses, that is, "the vital-qi is weak, and pathogenic factors invade into the human body". The deficiency of qi of the lung, spleen and kidney can all lead to weakness of lung-qi. Prolonged smoking creates heat that consumes body fluid, or excessive sexual intercourse consuming essence and blood can cause deficiency of lung-Yin, deficiency of Yin and internal heat, and deficiency of both qi and Yin. Exterior pathogenic factors can invade into the body as vital-qi is weakened. When pathogenic factors stay in the body, the movement of qi and circulation of blood is hindered. As the body fluid is not distributed, its accumulation turns into phlegm. This will cause phlegm and blood to come into contact with each other, finally forming a tumour after a long time. Hence, lung cancer is a local manifestation of disease of the whole body, and a disease due to deficiency, and excess syndrome due to deficiency. Deficiency syndrome in the early stage is mainly vital-qi of lung and spleen or the deficiency of both qi and Yin, and advanced lung cancer is mainly the deficiency of Yin and internal heat or the deficiency of both Yin and Yang. Local excess syndrome includes several pathological changes such as stagnation of qi, stasis of blood, coagulation of phlegm, and accumulation of toxin.

(b) Based on the theory of pathogenic toxin invading the lung, six exterior pathogenic factors invade the lung and cause dysfunction of dispersing and descending of the lung, stasis of lung-qi, obstruction of blood circulation, stagnation of qi and blood, and finally leading to tumour.

(c) Based on the theory of interior accumulation of phlegm and dampness, tumour is caused because of the deficiency of spleen and dysfunction of its transportation and transformation. This causes the accumulation of dampness and production of phlegm, and phlegm staying in the lung, stasis of lung-qi, dysfunction of dispersing and descending, coagulation of phlegm and accumulation of toxin.

Hong Guang-xiang (Hong, 1989) holds that in pathology, blood stasis is the basic pathogenesis in lung cancer, and blood stasis in lung is basic syndrome type. Chen Yu-kun (Chen, 1993) argues that phlegm and blood stasis are not only pathologic results due to pathogenic factors invading the lung and dysfunction of the viscera, but pathogenic factors can also lead to the internal deficiency of vital-qi, and the formation of tumour because of the combination of pathogenic factors and toxin. Hence, phlegm and blood stasis exist in the whole process of lung cancer. In conclusion, the cognition of aetiology and pathology of lung cancer tends to combine the theory of deficiency of vital-qi with the theory of pathogenic toxin, phlegm and blood stasis. In clinical treatment, the therapeutic effects are attained with the methods of combination of strengthening the body resistance, clearing away heat and toxic material, softening hard masses and resolving phlegm, and promoting blood circulation by removing blood stasis according to different syndromes.

7.3 Clinical Trial

7.3.1 *Study on therapeutic effect and its assessment standard*

At present, therapies for early- and middle-stage of lung cancer are mainly surgery, radiotherapy and chemotherapy, and the therapeutic effect can been improved with TCM. However, most patients are inoperable when diagnosed. Many clinical trials reported that quite a few patients in middle and advanced stage who are intolerable to radiotherapy and chemotherapy obtain a certain therapeutic effect in stabilising and decreasing focus, inhibiting infiltrating and metastasis, improving quality of life and prolonging survival period when they are treated with TCM. In recent years, according to statistical analysis of reports of therapeutic effects of treating over 100 advanced lung cancer patients with TCM only, stable rate of focus is about 67%–87% and median survival period is 9.5–13.8 months, which are better than the results in the control group treated by chemotherapy (Sun, 2000). In a clinical trial, Liu Jia-xiang (Liu *et al.*, 1995) reported on 304 cases of advanced lung cancer. The patients were randomly separated into TCM and chemotherapy groups. In the TCM group (171 cases), decreasing and stable rate (CR + PR + NC) was 67.83%; survival rates at one year, three years and five years were 60.94%, 31.86% and 24.22% respectively, and median survival period was 417 days. In the chemotherapy group (133 cases) treated with MOF regime at the corresponding period, decreasing and stable rate (CR + PR + NC) was 48.12%, survival rates at one year, three years and five years were 36.66%, 24.50% and 0%, respectively, and median survival period was 265 days. The rate of improvement of the clinical symptoms and the survival quality in the

TCM group are better than the chemotherapy group (Liu *et al.*, 1995). The therapeutic effect of treating lung cancer with TCM can be generalised as "living along with tumours". If local remission rate (CR or PR) of tumour is used for assessment standard of therapeutic effect only, the therapeutic effect of TCM would not be assessed completely. Chen Zhi-feng (Chen, 1996b) argues that the concept of tumour and the aim of treatment of tumour should be re-thought and re-understood. And using "living without tumours" as a standard of therapeutic effect is likely to cause excessive and unnecessary therapy. Liao Mei-ling (Liao, 1998) of Shanghai Chest Hospital designed an assessment table of life quality of lung cancer patient which includes 21 items and 84 markings. After primary assessment of 53 lung cancer cases treated with modern medical methods (surgery, chemotherapy and radiotherapy), she found that the marking of these patients decreased by 10.3, with the marking of patients treated with chemotherapy decreased by 7.5 on average, and the patients who got partial response (PR) decreased by 16 on average. So she concluded that the presently accepted assessment methods of therapeutic effect are only biological indexes that ignore other factors such as psychological, social, economic and individual differences. As a result, oncology scholars in China who study survival period and quality of life have paid more attention to the comprehensive therapies and the assessment standard of therapeutic effect that are suitable to the situation in China.

7.3.2 *Study on treatment based on syndrome differentiation*

In TCM, lung cancer is regarded as a local manifestation of systemic disease, and it should be treated by regulating the function of the human body from a holistic viewpoint, and treated with methods based on syndrome differentiation. This is because of the differences between prenatal heredity, age, process of disease, pathologic type, clinical stage and therapy method of different patients. Many obvious individual differences usually exist between patients, and this leads to different syndromes in the same disease. Hence, treatment based on syndrome differentiation is still used as a main therapeutic method in treating lung cancer with TCM, and is good for exploring the rules of diagnosis and treatment, and evaluating therapeutic effect.

Liu Jia-xiang (Liu *et al.*, 2001a and b) has reported the treatment of 310 cases of late lung cancer with TCM (treatment based on syndrome differentiation). All the cases were diagnosed by cytopathology, including 138 cases of squamous cell cancer, 80 cases of adenocarcinoma, 43 cases of undifferentiated cancer and 49 cases of unknown cytopathology. He divided these cases into five syndrome types according to syndrome differentiation: Yin-deficiency and internal heat, deficiency of both qi and Yin, deficiency of spleen and accumulation of phlegm and dampness, deficiency of both Yin and Yang, stagnation of qi and blood. Treatment was by the method of strengthening the body resistance, such as nourishing Yin to replenish fluid, supplementing qi and nourishing Yin, supplementing qi to strengthen spleen, nourishing Yin and warming Yang respectively, and combined with anti-tumour drugs that removes phlegm and softens hard masses, regulating the flow of qi and removing blood stasis, clearing heat and toxic material.

The survival rates of one, two, three and over five years after being treated with TCM alone were 43.23%, 11.3%, 5.2% and 0.2%, respectively. The longest survival period was 18 years, median survival period was 11.2 months and the average survival period was 12.6 months. In this group, the survival rates of one, two and three years of 64 adenocarcinoma cases after treatment were 35.94%, 11% and 4.6%, respectively.

Through statistical analysis of therapeutic effect, syndrome and pathologic types seem to be the more important factors that influence the prognosis than clinical stages, with syndrome type and clinical stage more closely related to recent therapeutic effect than pathologic type. Several indices of more than half of the patients after treatment obviously increased as compared to the state of pre-treatment ($P < 0.05$), including improvement of clinical symptom and immunologic indices such as phagocytosis function of phagocytes, transformational rate of lymphocytes and formational rate of E rosettes.

To verify the therapeutic effect of TCM, Liu *et al.* (2001a and b) studied 304 cases of late primary lung cancer (III, IV stage). The patients were randomly separated into TCM and chemotherapy groups (MOP). All 171 late primary adenocarcinoma of lung cancer cases in the TCM group were divided into four syndrome types: Yin-deficiency and internal heat; deficiency of both qi and Yin; deficiency of spleen and accumulation of phlegm and dampness; and deficiency of both Yin and Yang according to the syndrome type mentioned above. They were treated with drugs of strengthening the body such as nourishing Yin (upright ladybell root; fourleaf ladybell root, coastal glehnia root, cochinchinese asparagus root, dwarf lilyturf tuber, figwort root, lily bulb, rehmannia dride rhizome, shell of terrapin, etc.), supplementing qi (ginseng, tangshen, membranous milkvetch root, mongolian milkvetch root, heterophylly falsestarwort root, largehead atractylodes rhizome, india bread, etc.), warming Yang (malytea scurfpea fruit, korean epimedium herb, desert-living cistanche, dodder seed, songaroa cynomorium herb, fruit of climbing fig, etc.) respectively, and combined with drugs for removing phlegm and softening hard masses, clearing away heat and toxic material (common selfheal fruit-spike, seaweed, snakegourd peel, jackinthepulpit tuber, oyster shell, herb of Chinese Sage, spreading hedyotis herb, etc.).

Finally the decreasing rate of focus was 67.83%; survival rates of one, three and five years were 60.94%, 31.86% and 24.22%, respectively; median survival period was 11 months.

The improvement in life quality and immunologic function was overall better than that of the chemotherapy group, and good therapeutic effect was obtained.

Tang Wen-xiu divided lung cancer into four syndrome types: qi-deficiency of lung and spleen; deficiency of lung Yin; deficiency of both qi and Yin; and accumulation of phlegm and dampness and blood stasis. They were with modified Liu Jun Zi Decoction, Sha Shen Mai Dong Decoction, Sheng Mai Decoction, and Qian Jin Wei Jing Decoction respectively, combined with bistort rhizome, nightshade, spreading hedyotis herb, dandelion, baikal skullcap root, barbed skullcap herb, red root gromwel root, dried toad skin, leaf of fruticose dracaena, and Fei Liu Ping Gao, etc. 161 cases of advanced non-small cell lung cancer were treated by the method mentioned above. The result showed that the remission rate of tumour was 9.3%, and median survival period was 11 months, which is better than that of the chemotherapy group.

Cao Yang reported (Cao, 2000) that 31 cases of late NSCLC (6 cases were clinical diagnosis) were treated with syndrome differentiation, and the basic decoction is coastal glehnia root, cochinchinese asparagus root, chinese magnoliavine fruit, jackinthepulpit tuber, danshen root, common selfheal fruit-spike, hairyvein agrimonia herb, spreading hedyotis herb, etc. The result shows that PR was 9.7%, NC was 58.1%, median survival period was 10 months and the survival rates of one, two and three years were 32.3%, 7.2% and 3.6% respectively.

Fan Zong-ze (Fan, 1985) treated late lung adenocarcinoma according to the syndrome type of deficiency of both qi and Yin, deficiency of spleen and accumulation of phlegm and dampness, deficiency of both Yin and Yang, and compared the results with the chemotherapy control group. The stable and remission rate of tumour was no different between the two groups, but the average survival period of the TCM group was 330 days and the chemotherapy group was 143 days, showing an obvious difference between the two groups.

7.3.3 *Study on therapeutic principles and specific prescriptions*

The clinical syndrome type that occurs most frequently and the therapeutic principles and basic prescriptions (specific prescriptions) of lung cancer are summarised according to the clinical symptoms of lung cancer. This method of combining syndrome differentiation and disease differentiation is advantageous because it standardises clinical therapy and observation of therapeutic effect, which facilitates further study and exploitation of new drugs.

For example, Liu Jiu-xiang (Liu *et al.*, 1995) has statistically analysed TCM syndrome types of 310 cases of primary lung cancer and found that 80% of all cases (248 cases) pertained to the type of deficiency of both qi and Yin, and the type of Yin-deficiency and internal heat. Through many years of clinical trial and experimental research, he developed a new Chinese prescription: Yi Fei Kang Liu Yin (composed of membranous milkvetch root; mongolian milkvetch root, coastal glehnia root, cochinchinese asparagus root, glossy privet fruit, chinese paris rhizome, etc.), which mainly comprises of drugs for benefiting qi and nourishing Yin, combined with drugs for clearing heat and toxic material. One hundred and twenty-seven cases of NSCLC were treated by this new Chinese prescription, and the PR was 14 cases, NC was 89 cases, PD was 24 cases, rate of PR + NC was 81.10%, the survival rates of one, three and five years were 73.21%, 13.93% and 11.17% respectively, and the median survival period was 406 days. At the same time, 64 cases of lung cancer were treated by chemotherapy (MAP scheme), PR was 7 cases, NC was 39 cases, rate of PR + NC was 71.88%, the survival rates of one, three and five years were 40.54%, 11.06% and 5.53% respectively, and the median survival period was 267 days. The Yi Fei Kang Liu Yin group fared better than the chemotherapy group in the alleviation of symptoms, of health status and the improvement of immunologic indexes.

Wang Xi-ming (Wang, 1985) holds that the syndrome types of weakness of body resistance, deficiency of Yin and fluid and internal accumulation of pathogenic heat are frequently seen in lung cancer. He treated 50 cases of late lung cancer with Fu Zheng Yang Yin Tang (composed of rehmannia dride rhizome, cooked rehmannia dride rhizome, cochinchinese asparagus root, dwarf lilyturf tuber, figwort root; figwort, membranous milkvetch root; mongolian milkvetch root, tangshen, root of uniflower swisscentaury, rhizome of glabrous greenbrier, heartleaf houttuynia herb, skunk bugbane rhizome). The result showed that the survival rates of one, three and five years were 44%, 8% and 4% respectively.

Lin *et al.* (1998) reported that he treated 25 cases of NSCLC with Fu Fang Fei Liu Ping No. II (composed of membranous milkvetch root; mongolian milkvetch root, american ginseng, chinese paris rhizome, spreading hedyotis herb, peach seed, sanchi, etc.), and compared them with 10 cases treated by chemotherapy. The results showed that the effective rate of CR and PR of TCM group and chemotherapy group were 0 and 10% respectively, and the survival rate of one year was 28% and 10% respectively.

Chen Pei-feng (Chen, 1996a) treated 60 cases of late lung cancer with Yang Yin Qing Fei Tang (composed of upright ladybell root; fourleaf ladybell root, coastal glehnia root, dwarf lilyturf tuber, rehmannia dride rhizome, tree peony bark, fragrant solomonseal rhizome, snakegourd root, fig, etc.). The result showed that the survival rates of one and three years were 56.67% and 20%, respectively.

Wang *et al.* (1997) found that the syndrome type of deficiency of qi and blood stasis is 60.2% in all 108 cases of NSCLC, and treated them by strengthening qi, activating blood circulation and dispersing mass (membranous milkvetch root; mongolian milkvetch root, heterophylly falsestarwort root, coastal glehnia root, india bread; Tuckahoe, chinese magnoliavine fruit, common selfheal fruit-spike, common burreed rhizome, zedoary, sanchi, cattail pollen, herb of Chinese Sage, earthworm, etc.), with the combination of chemotherapy (CE or CAP scheme). The result was that the rate of PR and NC was 80.5%, the metastasis rate of 6 months was 29.3%, and the haemorrheologic indexes also showed certain improvement.

Wang Jin-rong (Wang, 1996) treated 64 cases of lung cancer by strengthening the body resistance and decreasing masses. The basic prescription is membranous milkvetch root; mongolian milkvetch root, tangshen, rehmannia dride rhizome, coix seed, danshen root, zedoary, agaric, glossy privet fruit, Pinellia tuber, caladium, heartleaf houttuynia herb, wasps nest, centipede, spreading hedyotis herb, barbed skullcap herb, etc. The result showed that the survival rates of one, two and three years were 46.9%, 45.6% and 7.8% respectively, and median survival period was 11 months.

7.3.4 *Study on new drugs and agents*

In the research on treatment of lung cancer, it is common to combine syndrome differentiation with disease differentiation, and to conduct studies on new Chinese drugs and agents that possess good therapeutic effect and are convenient for treatment. The new Chinese medicines, compound prescriptions and set prescriptions approved by the state include several new national Chinese medicine III such as Jin Fu Kang Oral Liquid, Fei Liu Ping Gao, etc. The Chinese anti-tumour drugs that are extracted from single Chinese herb and made into parenteral solution include Kang Lai Te Injection (extracted from coix seed), Lan Xiang Xi Injection (extracted from zedoray), Ya Dan Zi Emulsion, Ma Te Ling Injection (extracted from light yellow sophora root), Wei Mai Ning Capsule (extracted from wild rhizome of wild buckwheat), etc. These drugs have certain therapeutic effects when used in treating lung cancer.

7.3.5 *Study on therapy of combination of TCM and Western medicine*

Treating lung cancer with a combination of TCM and Western medicine can not only raise the inhibition rate of carcinoma, but also improve the status of body, decrease the side effects of radiotherapy and chemotherapy as well as prolong the survival period. Most studies show that this kind of therapy is better than radiotherapy or chemotherapy, especially in improving the median survival period.

For instance, Zhang Dai-zhao and Xu Jun-dong (Zhang and Xu, 1994) treated 36 cases of lung cancer with Fu Zheng Zeng Xiao Prescription (composed of membranous milkvetch root, largehead atractylodes rhizome, heterophylly falsestarwort root, barbary wolfberry fruit, suberect spatholobus stem, safflower, sappan wood, india bread; Tuckahoe, chicken gizzard membrane, dendrobium stem, coastal glehnia root, honeysuckle flower) 10 days prior to radiotherapy until the end of radiotherapy. The results were compared with another 35 cases treated by radiotherapy only. The result showed that the recent therapeutic effect (CR + PR) of the treatment group is 69.67%, higher than that of the control group. And the side effect observed in the treatment group is lower than that of the control group. Zhang concluded that treating lung cancer with traditional Chinese medicine and radiotherapy at the same time is a good method, and the traditional Chinese medicine contains drugs that can promote blood circulation and strengthen the body resistance.

Li Dao-yang (Li *et al.*, 2000) treated 61 cases of NSCLS with Fu Zheng Pai Du Kang Ai Prescription (composed of membranous milkvetch root, king solomonseal rhizome, ginseng, hairyvein agrimonia herb, heartleaf houttuynia herb, rhubarb, agaric, barbed skullcap herb, spreading hedyotis herb, jackinthepulpit tuber, Job's-tears, peach seed, snakegourd fruit, etc.) and chemotherapy at the same time, and comparing with the 61 cases treated by chemotherapy only. The result showed that the recent therapeutic effect (CR + PR) of the treatment group was 39.68%, while that of the control group was 25.49%. Also, the decrease of leucocyte and haemoglobin was better in the treatment group than in the control group.

Wang Xiao-ming and Xiong Mo-nian (Wang and Xiong, 1997) divided 50 cases into four types: the deficiency of both the lung and the spleen; the insufficiency of both qi and Yin; the accumulation of phlegm and dampness; and the stagnancy of qi and blood, and used Chinese drugs according to the above types. He treated the 50 cases of NSCLC with

Chinese drugs and chemotherapy (treated the adenocarcinoma with EP scheme, and squamous carcinoma with CAP scheme), and compared the results with the 30 cases treated by chemotherapy only. The results showed that the recent therapeutic effect (CR + PR + MR) of the treatment group was 42%, while that of the control group was 26%. The median survival period for the treatment group was 9 months while that of the control group was 3 months. The results of the treatment group were better than the control group in the improvement of symptoms and side effects.

Li Jin-han (Li, 1996) divided 102 cases randomly into two groups (groups A and B). He treated group A with Chinese drugs and chemotherapy, and group B with chemotherapy only. He divided group A into four types: the deficiency of both the lung and the spleen; the accumulation of phlegm and heat in the lung; the Yin deficiency of the lung and the stomach; and the stagnancy of qi and blood, and used Chinese drugs according to the above types. He treated the SCLC with EP scheme of chemotherapy, and NSCLC with CTPC scheme of chemotherapy. The result showed that the recent therapeutic effect (CR + PR) of group A is 52.1%, group B is 35.2% (comparison of the two groups, $P > 0.05$). The survival rate of one year in group A was 69.4%, and that of group B was 66.7% ($P < 0.05$). The median survival period of group A was 13 months, and that of group B was 9 months. The results showed that combining TCM and Western medicine can prolong survival period.

Chu Da-tong (Chu, 1998) divided 80 cases into two groups: one treated with chemotherapy (MVP) and Kang Lai Te injection, and the other with chemotherapy (MVP) only. The result showed that the recent therapeutic effect (CR + PR) of the former was 45%, and that of the latter was 22%. There is a significant discrepancy between the two groups.

Liu *et al.* (2001a and b) reported the results of the stage II clinical trial of the new Chinese drug Jin Fu Kang Oral Liquid. He divided 190 cases into two groups: one that was treated with chemotherapy (MVP or CAP) and Jin Fu Kang Oral Liquid, and the other one with chemotherapy (MVP or CAP) only. The results showed that the recent therapeutic effect (CR + PR) of the former was 42%, that of the latter was 23.33%. There is a significant discrepancy between the two groups ($P < 0.05$). The results of two clinical trial above showed that the therapeutic effect of NSCLC can be raised significantly by using Kang Lai Te injection or Jin Fu Kang Oral Liquid with chemotherapy.

Liu *et al.* (1995) treated 80 cases of NSCLC with the Chinese drug Lung-Nourishing Anti-Tumour Beverage and chemotherapy (MAP scheme), and treated another 64 cases with chemotherapy only. The results showed that the recent therapeutic effect (CR + PR) of the former was 87.5%, and that of the latter was 71.88%. Liu *et al.* observed the status of long distant metastases (to lung, liver, bone, brain, pericardium, pleura, suprarenal gland, subcutaneous part, etc.) of stage III lung cancer cases after treatment, and the result showed that the rate of long distant metastasis of the group treated with Yi Fei Kang Liu Yin and chemotherapy (85 cases) was 23.52%, and the group treated with only chemotherapy (42 cases) was 35.7%. The Yi Fei Kang Liu Yin has an effect to the anti-metastasis of lung cancer significantly.

7.4 The Experience and Future Prospects

In the recent 20 years, the experience in treating lung cancer with TCM and a combination of TCM and Western medicine showed the effectiveness of TCM. In aetiology factor and pathogenesis, several theories have been put forward, such as the Weakened Body Resistance, Pathogenic Poison, Blood Stasis, etc. with corresponding prescriptions and drugs. In clinical trials, the theories of TCM are used to guide diagnosis and treatment based on overall analysis of symptoms and signs, the cause, nature and location of the illness and the patients' physical condition. Most scholars think that lung cancer is a kind of syndrome of deficiency in origin and excess in superficiality, and they combine the theory of Weakened Body Resistance with the theory of Pathogenic Poison, Phlegm and Blood Stasis.

They treat lung cancer mainly by strengthening the body resistance combined with methods of clearing away heat and toxic material, softening hard masses, and resolving phlegm, or promoting blood flow. These therapeutic methods can raise therapeutic effect.

According to TCM theory, the aetiological factor and pathogenesis of occurrence and progress of lung cancer is a complicated biological process related to many factors and systems. And the treatment of lung cancer is based on the concept of holism, the rule of diagnosis and treatment based on overall analysis of symptoms and signs, the combination of diagnosis based on disease and symptoms, the combination of strengthening the body resistance and elimination of the pathogenic factor, and comprehensive consideration from multi-targets. This is one of the typical therapeusis of lung cancer of TCM in China.

The results of treatment of lung cancer with TCM is characterised by the high stable rate of focus, long survival period, good quality of life, and having potential superiority in resistance of relapse and metastasis. Therefore the remission rate of local focus alone cannot signify the traits of therapeutic effect of TCM. It can objectively show the therapeutic effect of TCM if following factors are taken into consider-ation: the remission rate (CR + PR) of tumour, the stable rate (PR + NR), long survival rate, average survival period, median survival period, quality of life, etc.

The aim of treatment of malignant tumour is to prolong the survival period and improve the quality of life of patients. Studies should be further conducted to classify the types of syndromes, and study the essence of these syndromes. The theoretical and technological development of modern pathology, biochemistry, immunology and molecular biology will provide better conditions for studying the types of syndromes and the mechanism of treating tumours with TCM objectively and at microcosmic level.

The increased therapeutic effect of treating lung cancer is a significant development that will enrich modern oncology. Furthermore, in recent years, some scholars have analysed symptoms of lung cancer and the frequency of drug use, selected effective drugs in order to form basic prescription or produce new agents based on clinical therapeutic effect, conduct clinical trials or experiments of pharmacodynamics, and assess the therapeutic effect. These studies will develop more safe and effective new drugs of TCM. This will also help develop methods of diagnosis and treatment based on overall analysis of symptoms and signs, the cause, nature and location of the illness and the patients' physical conditions according to the basic theories of traditional Chinese medicine, and improve the level of diagnosis and treatment of TCM and combination of TCM and Western medicine to reform Chinese drugs and develop new drugs of TCM.

References

Cao, Y., Li, Z., He, X.L., *et al.* (2000) Treating 31 cases of non-small cell lung cancer with differentiation of symptoms and signs. *J. Beijing Univ. Tradit. Chin. Med.* **23**(2), 66.

Chen, P.F. (1996a) Clinical report on treating 60 cases of late pulmonary carcinoma with Yang Yin Qing Fei Tang. *J. Sichuan Tradit. Chin. Med.* **14**(6), 20.

Chen, Y.K. (1993) The theory and clinical use of the therapeutical method of resolving phlegm and removing blood stasis. *New J. Tradit. Chin. Med.* **25**(1), 10–12.

Chen, Z.F. (1996b) Re-recognition of the conception of tumor and speculation on research of treatment with TCM. *Chin. J. Integr. Chin. West. Med.* **16**(6), 368–370.

Chu, D.T. (1998) *Proceedings of Studies on Anti-tumor of Kang Lai Te*. The Publishing Company of Zhejiang University, China, p. 192.

Fan, Z.Z. (1985) Clinical observation of late primary adenocaricinoma of lung treated by method of TCM. *Chin. J. Integr. Chin. West. Med.* **8**, 25–26.

Hong, G.X. (1989) Experience on treatment of primary late pulmonary carcinoma with TCM. *Chin. J. Tradit. Clin. Med. Pharm.* **4**(6), 42–43.

Li, D.Y., Ou, C.M., Li, G.D., *et al.* (2000) Clinical observation of Fu Zheng Bai Du Kang Ai prescription in action of raising therapeutic effect and relieving side effect of chemotherapy of non-small cell lung cancer. *Chin. J. Integr. Chin. West. Med.* **20**(3), 208–209.

Li, D.P. (1998) *Proceedings of Studies on Anti-tumour of Kang Lai Te*. The Publishing Company of Zhejiang University, p. 192.

Li, J.H. (1996) Clinical observation on treatment of pulmonary carcinoma with the method of combination of TCM and chemotherapy. *Chin. J. Integr. Chin. West. Med.* **16**(3), 136–138.

Li, L.D., Lu, F.Z., Zhang, S.W., *et al.* (1997) Analyses of variation trend and short term detection of Chinese malignant tumour mortality during twenty years. *Chin. J. Oncol.* **19**(1), 3.

Liao, M.L. (1998) *Contemporary Therapy of Lung Cancer*. The Publishing Company of Shanghai Medical University, Shanghai, pp. 364–368.

Lin, H.S., Li, S.Q., Pu, B.K., *et al.* (1998) The study on action of compound prescription of Chinese drug on anti-tumour and anti-metastasis of patient of lung cancer. *Chin. J. Surg. Integr. Tradit. Chin. West. Med.* **4**(5), 277–279.

Liu, J.X., Shi, Z.M., Xu, Z.Y., *et al.* (1995) Studies on late primary adenocarcinoma of lung treated by methods of nourishing-Yin to replenish fluid and warming-Yang to benefit qi. *J. Tradit. Chin. Med.* **36**(3), 155–157.

Liu, J.X. (1996) *The Big System of Modern Application and Study of TCM Vol. 14*. The Section of Oncology. The Publishing Company of Shanghai University of TCM, Shanghai.

Liu, J.X., Pan, M.Q., Li, Y.H., *et al.* (2001a) Clinical study of Jin Fu Kang oral liquid for treating NSCLC. *Tumour* **21**(6), 463–464.

Liu, J.X., Shi, Z.M., Li, H.G., *et al.* (2001b) Clinical observation of "lung-nourishing anti-tumour beverage" in treating non-small cell lung cancer in 271 cases. *Shanghai J. Tradit. Chin. Med.* **2**, 4–6.

Sun, G. (2000) Advancement and speculation on TCM treatment of lung cancer. *Jiangsu J. Tradit. Chin. Med.* **21**(1), 44.

Wang, J.R. (1996) Treatment of 64 cases of pulmonary carcinoma with principle of strengthening the body resistance and decreasing masses. *Liaoning J. Tradit. Chin. Med.* **23**(11), 495–496.

Wang, X. and Xiong, M.N. (1997) Treating 50 cases of late non-small cell lung cancer with combination of TCM and Western medicine. *Chin. J. Surg. Integr. Tradit. Chin. West. Med.* **3**(2), 98–99.

Wang, X.M. (1985) Treating primary bronchogenic carcinoma with the methods of strengthening the body resistance and nourishing Yin to replenish fluid. *Liaoning J. Tradit. Chin. Med.* **8**, 25–26.

Wang, X.M., Yu, R.C., Wang, Y.T., *et al.* (1997) Clinical study on treating late non-small cell lung cancer with the methods of benefiting qi, promoting blood circulation, dissolving lumps and chemotherapy. *Chin. J. Integr. Chin. West. Med.* **17**(2), 86–87.

Zhang, D.Z. and Xu, J.D. (1994) Clinical and experimental study of Fu Zheng Zeng Xiao prescription on action of improving the effect of body resistance. *Chin. J. Integr. Chin. West. Med.* **14**(9), 561–562.

Chapter 8

Direction of TCM Modernisation and Quality Control Mode

Pei-shan Xie & Eric Wong

Abstract

In the past 50 years, China has made gigantic steps towards the proper control of herbal products. The work on quality control at this stage, has branched out into: (1) single entity extraction type of products and (2) traditional formulation products. Although extractions do possess successful examples, e.g. artemisinin and taxol, they do not represent Chinese medicine as it exists conventionally. Such endeavours, by the way, have been extremely difficult and costly. The traditional formulation products, on the other hand, are consistent with conventional teachings. As long as herb traders respect research and clinical trials, objective evidences will be worked out on their efficacy, which will lead the way towards the modernisation of Chinese medicine in this era of globalisation. The example of research on Gingko leaves is a good illustration to the fallacy of insistence on single-active compound. Scientists engaged in Gingko research, on the contrary, realised that total group compounds and active fractions served better to give therapeutic explanation to the efficacy than the assumption of a single compound. The concept of multiple constituents being responsible for the efficacy rather than a single active compound has been endorsed by the WHO and has become the acceptable focus of research on herbal preparations. In the thorough quality control of herbal preparations, different forms of finger printing records should be established.

Keywords: Chinese Medicine; Herbal Products; Quality Control.

After a half-century under strict governmental control, the development of traditional Chinese medicine (TCM) has made giant leaps towards modernisation with enormous achievements. A country's policy of openness presents an opportunity to promote the age-old truths of natural healing through TCM. The current trend of TCM modernisation is a welcome new wave in this cold modern world of high-speed technology and higher-speed information.

The definite course and development of TCM can be traced in the modernisation of TCM quality control, efficacy/toxicology of TCM and the modernisation of the TCM industry — of which two branches have evolved:

(1) *Single-entity-mining type TCM products:* These comprise of a single active constituent isolated, characterised chemically and pharmacologically from Chinese herbal drugs. Originally derived from the traditional use of TCM, the isolation of the active constituent separates itself from TCM philosophy and practice. As a single entity, it is generally better accepted by Western thinkers and the Western system [often erroneously touted as the only scientific approach (Leung, 2002)], but has little or no relation to TCM. In the past century, researchers everywhere have made painstaking efforts to isolate and characterise the "active constituent(s)" in botanicals or other natural resources, which have proven to be successful. Prime examples include: artemisinin and taxol. Without doubt, this form of research approach will continue to be popular, especially in exploring a novel "active constituent" from a new source of origin such as the marine ecosystem, or modifying the chemical structure from an existing single active component to enhance its efficacy and/or reduce its toxicity).

To contemplate the past century, however, the fact is clear that only a few single active compounds from natural resources were recognised unanimously and approved officially as pharmaceuticals, although hundreds and thousands components were excessively isolated from herbal drugs through generations' efforts. The low benefits and high risks for mining novel single active compounds from herbal drugs should be seriously considered. The "single-entity-mining" model is not suitable for the purposes of TCM philosophy and will ultimately be insufficient to fully characterise TCM. Moreover, researchers and manufacturers of TCM should consider the many drawbacks including financial and technological disadvantages and limits in using the Western system with TCM.

(2) *"Herbal-intact-retaining" type TCM products:* In keeping with historical/empirical formulation combined with modern-day processes and dosage forms, the traditional characteristic of original TCM doctrine is basically held. This "herbal-intact-retaining" approach may seem difficult to grasp by Western logic. There is the unfamiliar feature rooted from the holistic efficacy of multiple actives and unknown active components, and the unique but abstruse philosophy of TCM being used in TCM clinical practice. Cultural and historical sameness may pose hindrances to Westerners in unraveling the secrets of TCM. It would be an unforgivable tragedy to damage the reputation of TCM philosophy simply because of greed, ignorance and lack of in-depth investigations during the development of such a TCM industry which focuses only on making a quick-profit.

Although the two branches have fundamental differences in research model and methodologies, both share the common goal of identifying potential uses of TCM in disease prevention, health promotion and increasing longevity. The final outcome of unifying both "orthodox" medicines with Chinese medicine into one universally accepted practice of medicine will eventually be reached but not without an extensive period of research and practical studies. The pace at which this ideal system is achieved will largely depend on how TCM knowledge is shared.

TCM philosophy is very difficult to describe and explain in modern scientific terms for wide acceptance and understanding. Therefore evidence collected and proven over thousands of years of Chinese history must not be so quickly discarded. The responsibility should reasonably fall on the shoulders of today's generation who are educated and cultured in the environment of Chinese culture as well as modern scientific knowledge.

Success in the course of TCM modernisation relies heavily upon the proper allocation of time, respect and resource to scientifically understand TCM philosophy. Such efforts will be futile if inherent cultural awareness is weak, or language barriers exist, or both. For these reasons, TCM promotion is a challenging endeavour for us. It is therefore critical, from the very beginning, to concentrate on the clear interpretation of TCM philosophy with modern scientific methods and with a language of general acceptance.

It is interesting to note that the findings of a German study performed on *Gingko biloba* leaves coincide with TCM clinical experience. With thorough comprehensive research and extensive data collection, the findings of this German study have achieved international acclaim. (In contrast, 1000-year-old TCM philosophies have yet to be proven or described in a manner for popular acceptance.) After 30 years of research on the active constituents of Gingko leaf extract, the German group appointed the total flavonoids and total terpene lactones as active fractions to represent the efficacy of Gingko leaves rather than assigning it to any single component. Abandoning the single-active-constituent approach was not due to their technical unfeasibility, instead it was based on many years of research that the following conclusions were arrived: (1) The pharmacological activity of Gingko leaves is not fully understood; (2) strong activity has been linked to both Ginkgo total flavonoids and total terpene lactones; and (3) other constituents, not showing any activity alone, may contribute to the total efficacy since their removal from the extract resulted in lower efficacy.

These scientific findings have suggested the concept of "multi-components" contributing to total herb efficacy, and that they are in compliance with TCM clinical practice and its holistic philosophy. The difference in general acceptance rests on the fact that the German findings are supported by scientific data with control while TCM hypotheses are lacking in support of modern scientific evidence. Furthermore, the massive amount of data accumulated by German scientists has allowed them to address all issues of pharmacological importance and clinical safety relating to Gingko leaves. Regrettably, this very ancient Chinese medicinal herb was rarely acknowledged as such, and throughout the years *Ginkgo biloba* was never recorded in any Chinese Herbal Compendium. (Its exclusion may have been due to toxic Ginkgolic acids contained in Ginkgo leaves which could not be removed in aqueous decoctions without any pre-treatment.) The German study should be used as a reference for TCM research, to apply theoretical and practical aspects of TCM whilst retaining its philosophy. However, this resource-consuming and time-intensive approach, with little short-term financial return is not of particular interest to most of the Chinese medicine industry.

In a World Health Organization (WHO) West Pacific Regional Meeting, a draft of *Strategic Plan for Regional Traditional Medicine* pointed out that "There are many challenges facing standardisation of traditional medicine practice and products. For example, herbal medicines differ from chemical synthetic drugs in several very important ways. Herbal medicines usually contain numerous chemical compounds rather than a single active compound. Often, not all active components of herbal medicines have been isolated, characterised or quantified. The efficacy of a medicinal plant or mixture of several plants is the result of the pharmacological activity of a blend of one or more species of herb. Even a single plant is not a purified simple chemical compound. Standard techniques for the control of individual purified components may not be applicable to complex herbal medicines, requiring some modifications to existing regulatory systems. Collaboration among countries in the region will be needed if regulatory standards govern herbal medicine" (WHO, 2001). This concept of "multi-constituent" contribution to herbal efficacy is well accepted by many countries and the WHO. Among many countries practicing their own traditional medicine, TCM is the only one supported by a systematic and comprehensive theory and practical system. Therefore, it will be a great loss for the human race if TCM does not undergo the thorough and proper scientific investigation that it deserves.

Whichever model is utilised in the modernisation of TCM industry, proper quality control measures in TCM are essential for its further advancement. The "single-active-constituent" QC model is solidly established in the chemical pharmaceutical industry. However, this model applies poorly in the control of the quality of TCM, which shows efficacy in the "multi-component" environment. Perhaps it would be more appropriate to apply similar QC measures from the food, wine or perfume industries to herbal drug quality control. The characteristic taste of wines or the special scent of perfumes is attributed to its "multi-component" fraction, not to any single component. For example, there are yearly variations in the flavour and aroma of different brands of whisky. The combination of gas chromatography with aromatic analysis is employed to confirm the mixture of a group of components with relative consistent proportion and concentration. Realistically, the TCM industry must be equally, if not more, discriminating. The efficacy of TCM is based on the collaboration, antagonism and synergism of its multi-components, to reach a macro-governance status. Thus, it is necessary to develop a type of QC system to be able to meet the complex, non-linear, comprehensive characteristics of TCM. To date, the new QC mode — the chromatographic fingerprinting analysis — is the best possible solution for application of herbal quality control (Xie, 2001). It utilises chromatographic methods to achieve an overall quality assessment. The entire chromatogram's characteristic is under evaluation, not any particular component, peak, or pin-point. Rather, the wholeness of the profile is emphasised and is significance for the total quality information it represents.

At present, the State Food and Drug Administration (SFDA) in China has requested for the manufacturers of TCM herbs (of the injectable dosage form) to disclose a Fingerprinting Profile as part of its product specifications. The practice of fingerprinting provides a marco-analytical approach to evaluate the quality of the product and to identify any adulterants. Furthermore, the fingerprinting analysis supplies quantifiable information to evaluate the suitability of the processing procedures, product stability and quality consistency.

Fingerprinting is a sustainable quality control mode for TCM. Through active research and with rapid development in both analytical techniques and computer capacity, the fingerprinting analysis will be constantly improved and fine-tuned. In addition, this QC mode is complementary with findings from areas of pharmacology, biochemistry, clinical research and TCM philosophy. A system to correlate fingerprinting data with the TCM efficacy can be expected in the future. Eventually, a relationship can be elucidated between a characterised fingerprinting profile and its corresponding herb/formulation efficacy. This would be the ultimate goal for developing the fingerprinting technique. However, it is important to recognise that the fingerprinting analysis also has its limitations.

Particularly for herbs, the active principles cannot be totally detected by the current chromatographic techniques. And the uncertainty in the presence or activity of certain constituents within TCM may cause inconsistencies in fingerprinting results and affect its relationship with efficacy. (These uncertainties are also problematic in clinical evaluations.) And there may be other unforeseeable questions or difficulties in the usage of fingerprinting technique in the development process that need to be conquered. Nevertheless, the wholeness-targeted quality assessment mode achieved by fingerprinting analysis will advance the quality control of TCM forward another progressive step in its continual development and modernisation.

In closing, keeping the concepts of "decomposition" and "accuracy" in mind and firmly under a conventional analytical chemistry atmosphere, most herbal analysts consider it is confusing and unacceptable when the aspects of "wholeness" and "uncertainty" are integral in quality control of TCM through chromatographic fingerprinting. It is therefore very important to realise that a change at the conceptual level is essential when abandoning the well-accepted QC mode for chemical pharmaceutical for a more proper QC mode — the fingerprinting analysis that better meets the needs of TCM. A shift in paradigm is needed to access this new arena. And other scientific disciplines, namely biochemistry, chemometrics and computer science, will definitely be employed and merged to strengthen and support the development of TCM fingerprinting analysis, as it will to analytical chemistry.

References

Leung, A.Y. (2002) What's lacking in peer-reviewed publications? *Leung's (Chinese) Herb News*, March/April, No. 37, AYSL Corporation, USA (ISSN# 1523-5017).

World Health Organization (WHO) (2001) WPR/RC52/7: *A Draft Regional Strategy for Traditional Medicine in Western Pacific*. WHO Regional Committee, 52nd session, Brunei Darussalam, 10–14 September.

Xie, P. (2001) A feasible strategy for applying chromatographic fingerprint to assess quality of Chinese herbal medicine. In: *Proceedings of International Symposium of Quality Assessment of TCM by Chromatographic Fingerprint*, Guangzhou, China, 20–21 February, pp. 40–56 (revised version).

Chapter 9

A Critical Look at Traditional Medicine Recommendations in the Line of Research Approach

Ping-chung Leung

Abstract

While full recognition of the Practical Value of Traditional Chinese Medicine is being endorsed, the current stand on the Research Methodology of this field should be worked out. Since modern medicine has already developed a logical system of research methodology basing on the principles of deduction, any research on any system of medicine need to take reference to what is most popularly used and commonly recommended. The best way to approach research on Chinese Medicine, therefore, would be one that would take full reference to the methodology being used in modern medicine. This would enable traditional medicine to be elevated to the level of modern practice. Nevertheless, innate problems in traditional medicine are making its research difficult. The problems lie in the difficulties to achieve uniform herb supply, randomisation, placebo arrangement, uncertain chemical structures and toxicology, etc. A practical approach centered on carefully planned evidence-based clinical trials, with parallel studies on biological activities and herb authentication is being recommended.

Keywords: Chinese Medicine: Research Methodology: Evidence-Based Medicine.

9.1 Introduction

While modern medicine has offered a lot to mankind and is still advancing at fast speed which is beyond our imagination many years ago, alternative methods of treatment are still gaining much support and popularity

(Hannallah *et al.*, 2002; Lieberman *et al.*, 2002; Eisenberg and Roger, 1998). In the past decade, both clinicians and patients adopted a realistic attitude towards alternative medicine. They wanted to know more about the true efficacy of alternative medicine so that it can be used as an alternative treatment option. Users of Traditional Medicine (a form of complementary alternative medicine [TM-CAM]) may have a much more committed attitude as they were more culturally influenced (Klemman, 1975; Ayurveda Medicine, 2000). However, the quest for more evidence on the effectiveness of the traditional treatment has also taken a renewed importance (Goldbeck *et al.*, 1996; Kaptchuk and Eisenberg, 1998).

9.2 Evidence on the Efficacy of TM-CAM

9.2.1 *History of TM-CAM*

Traditional Medicine can be traced back for at least over 2500 years — this was proved in excavations which revealed prescriptions in various carvings and ancient metal or bamboo acupuncture needles. The numerous volumes of well written texts on the art of healing were remarkable, and showed that proper medical documentation started as early as 2000 BC. The study of infectious disease was documented in the Han Dynasty (Zhang Zhong Jieng), medical ethics was discussed in the Tang Dynasty (Suen Tse-Miu) and forensic medicine developed in the Sung Dynasty (Sung Tse). There were also special volumes discussing about pulses (Mijing) and difficult cases (Nianjing). It is widely agreed that of the many systems of ancient medicine, Chinese Medicine possessed the most sophisticated philosophy and literature, even though other systems of TM-CAM had equally lengthy histories.

9.2.2 *Archives on TM-CAM*

A survey was done in 2002 on the circulating journals in China pertaining to Chinese Medicine. The results were as follows:

(i) Total number of Chinese journals on Traditional Chinese Medicine (TCM) research (Chinese Medicine Med-line)

Category	Number
Chinese Medicine	89
Chinese-Western, Integrated Medicine	16
Herbs, Acupuncture, Manual Therapy, etc.	40

(ii) New Chinese journals on TCM research (Chinese Medicine Med-line)

Year of publication: 50s — 12; 60s — 0; 70s — 12;
80s — 53; 90s — 34; 2000 — 10

(iii) New subject areas in 2000 — Herbal drugs: 3

(New Journals)	Diet supplement	1
	Massage	1
	Health promotion	2
	Herbal Science	1
	Review	2

The statistics showed that there has been a real, increasing interest on Traditional Chinese Medicine in China and we can look forward to more modern utilisations, adaptations and research on Chinese Medicine (Cheng, 2001; Lai, 2002).

9.2.3 *Current modern literature*

Less than a decade ago, we saw a new journal appearing in China, titled *Chinese Journal of Integrated Traditional and Western Medicine*. Since then, more and more English language journals began accepting research articles related to Chinese Medicine. To quote one example, the *Journal of American Medical Association* had one special issue in 1999 that was dedicated to alternative medicine, and 70% of the articles were on acupuncture or Chinese Medicine (Eisenberg, 1998).

Indeed, the interest of consumers on alternative medicine and "off-the-counter" preparations in drug stores, has been well reflected by the number of scientific articles appearing in various well established journals, which traditionally have not been supportive on research areas considered to be "unscientific". In the recent SARS outbreak, the *Lancet* published a remarkable report from Germany, stating the *in vitro* effects of a root extract, glycyrrhizin, in the control of replication of SARS associated coronavirus (Cinatl *et al.*, 2003). This is a good example of the increasing attention being paid to Chinese Medicine, which obviously will lead to more scientific research.

9.2.4 *Current practices*

If modern medicine is perfect in the identification of the causes of diseases, their courses of events and subsequent effective treatment, there would be no place for TM-CAM. However, there are areas where the exact aetiology, pathological changes and subsequent management, are not yet clear. Therefore, the outcomes in these areas become uncertain.

There are plenty of examples: viral infections, allergic conditions, degenerative diseases, chronic problems, aging and cancer. Patients who get disappointed with modern treatments frequently go for TM-CAM treatment as a supplement or substitution. It is not uncommon to see satisfactory results from such treatment.

We cannot rely on such positive observations to establish the efficacy of TM-CAM. However, such observations should serve to encourage serious research on TM-CAM.

9.2.5 *Herb-derived pharmaceuticals*

Research on Herbal Medicine in the past century has been focused on many aspects: from pharmacocognosy, quality control, to authentication and clinical uses. Of these approaches, much resources have been spent on attempts to identify the active principles and working out the chemical formula with the obvious intension of developing an effective drug. There are a few successful examples in and outside China. One remarkable successful attempt in China was achieved through research efforts on the herbal treatment for malaria. Derivatives of Artemisinin (Qinghao) have, apart from successfully developed into an effective anti-malarial drug, recently been found to be also effective against some other parasites and certain cancers (Valecha and Tripath, 1997).

Two successful examples outside China would be vincristine and vinblastin, extracted from the flower periwinkle and taxol from the bark of Yew trees. All these pharmaceuticals are cytotoxic drugs that are produced in the National Chemistry Laboratory of France (CNRS, 1999).

Although current successful examples have been few, they do provide solid evidence that TM could develop into efficacious pharmaceuticals.

9.3 Major Challenges to the Evidence of Efficacy of TM-CAM

9.3.1 *Past archives might not be reliable*

While history provides macroscopic guidelines, it is unable to dictate what can be accepted today and what needs to be done.

Although past and current literature is available, it may not be practically and scientifically reliable.

In 1997, the Centre for the Promotion of Chinese Culture in Hong Kong organised a contest which asked for submission of scientific manuscripts pertaining to research on Chinese Medicine. Over 10,000 entries were submitted and these could be categorized into three main groups: viz., clinical studies (6090); laboratory work (3403); and analysis on Chinese Medicine Classics (1435). Ten experts from China and five Hong Kong scholars were responsible for the evaluation. The results were quite disappointing as the best quality papers came from the Chinese Medicine Classics group, whilst laboratory research reports were rather narrow in scope and superficial; and clinical studies did not follow the rules of evidence-based medicine (Leung and Wong, 2002).

In 1987, Tang *et al.* (1999) examined publications on Chinese Medicine and found that most of them failed to reach the quality required within the realm of meta-analysis. Fundamental requirements in case selection, randomisation, blinding techniques, use of placebo and quality control, were not well observed.

9.3.2 *Clinical efficacy needs to be proven with modern methodology*

The standard methodology for the test of efficacy is the conduction of a clinical trial based on good clinical practice. The most acceptable format would be a randomised control trial with double blinding and placebo.

However, the use of such logical methodology for TM-CAM research will result in more difficulties when compared with other clinical research situations.

(a) Clinical uniformity

Firstly, case selection is not straightforward. Case selection should be done according to strict criteria. However, when practitioners of Chinese Medicine are partners of the research, they emphasise on symptomatology rather than the diagnosis of the disease entity; syndrome presentation rather than investigations on the pathology. The tendency of the traditional practitioner to change the treatment modality according to changing behaviour is another unfavourable factor towards uniformity.

(b) Randomisation

Secondly, randomisation is not easy. Clients who come for treatment usually carry a strong intention for immediate treatment using Chinese Medicine. They tend to have this subjective demand because they either have had a bad experience with modern medicine or they have been influenced, socially or culturally, to take a positive view on Chinese Medicine. Persuading such individuals to accept the randomisation process would not be easy.

(c) Placebos

Thirdly, placebo arrangement is difficult. The Chinese patients are particularly against the use of placebo for the same reasons as randomisation. To produce physically identical preparations is also difficult when one insists not only on shape, size, colour and texture, but also on taste and smell.

(d) Uniform drugs

Uniformity of drugs can be achieved only through a uniform manufacturing process of a uniform chemical compound with a known chemical equation. When the chemical equation is unknown and even the active principles are not known, it is very often not possible to attain uniformity.

(e) Terminology of herbs

The lack of uniformity exists not only in the cultivation and harvests of herbs, but also in the basic identification of herbs, which could be divergent in some special areas. For instance, some herbs are functionally labeled, and many different botanical types could have been labeled as such, although they have nothing similar botanically. Tougucao (meaning: bone penetrating weed), a commonly used herb for bone injuries, owns 22 different botanical entities (Yu and Boa, 2000).

(f) Toxicity

Another problem is herb toxicity. Reports are rising on areas of life-threatening toxicity, e.g. against liver and kidney. The most common ones are those involving heavy metals and contaminants. Adverse effects not amounting to toxicity are subtle and even more dangerous because of their hidden nature and possibly wide implications (Suen *et al.*, 1998). As more and more food supplements and supplementary health promotion items of botanical origins appear in the market, there is a growing concern of possible interaction between these health promotion agents and the standard modern medicine that the majority of senior citizens are actually consuming. If someone is taking food supplements for cancer, will the supplement interfere with what he is receiving for treatment? If a supplement is being given to lower the dependence on steroid, will it interfere with the action of steroid? (De Smet and Accy, 1996) Many such questions need to be answered.

(g) Acupuncture

In acupuncture, it is even more difficult when a placebo is insisted upon. Although many suggestions and modalities of placebo puncture have been practiced and reported, including sham site (intentionally avoiding the correct sites of acupuncture points), sham punctures (scratching, superficial entry, enter and withdraw, touches, etc.), and specially manufactured needle with sham device, none of these fulfill the strict criteria required for a placebo. Moreover, the recipients' ignorance could be satisfactory in a short time, but with repeated punctures, they would learn to detect the differences. When electrical stimulation is used in addition to the puncture, placebo becomes totally impossible (Streitberge and Kleinhenz, 1998; Vincent and Lewith, 1995).

9.4 Setting Up a System of Research for Evidence-Based Efficacy of TM-CAM

After a brief review on the promises and difficulties of TM-CAM, it must be clear now that a direction could be set for a system of research for the evidence-based efficacy of TM-CAM.

9.4.1 *Set the priority areas*

One should selectively choose priority areas where modern medicine has not yet found perfect solutions. Priority areas include allergy, viral infection, cancer, degenerative diseases, ageing and preventive measures. These are the areas that research on TM-CAM offers great potential for supplementary solutions to unsolved clinical problems.

9.4.2 *The efficacy driven approach*

Pharmacocognosy — the field of identifying the active principles from the herbs and working out the chemical equation — is the most scientific way of developing herbal medicine. However, this is a lengthy, expensive way and there have been only few successes in the recent past. There is a compromise. The compromise aims at proving the efficacy of the raw herbal material or raw formula of herbs, before considering further sophisticated analysis. This is much less expensive and less time-consuming compared with the conventional method. This approach could be represented diagrammatically as in Fig. 9.1.

The Centre of Research is the clinical trial which is targeting an important clinical problem which fails to find a perfect solution in modern medicine. Choosing a methodology of universally high quality for the clinical trial would enable the results of the trial to be widely accepted, thus convincing the clinical experts on the efficacy of the

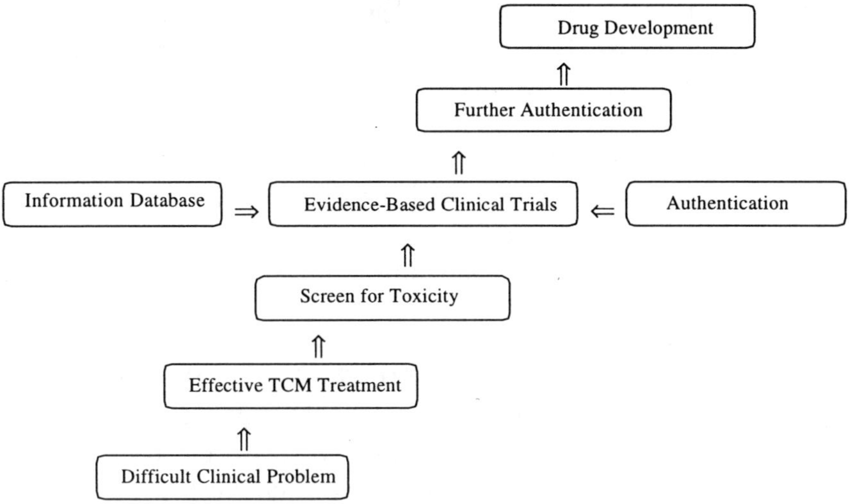

Figure 9.1. The efficacy driven approach.

treatment modality. Efficacy is most important to the clinician. Efficacy, once proven, encourages more utilisation and invites more commitments on further studies towards further improvement of the drug preparation.

Once efficacy is proven and determination is made towards further research, the following principles are enforced:

(a) *Understand the details of clinical influences*

Efficacy is taken as a macroscopic, crude demonstration of the effects of the modality of treatment used for a clinical problem. Once preliminary evidences are established, more details of the clinical influences could be worked out.

(b) *Understand the mode of action of the herbal formula*

This mainly involves laboratory tests, including animal models and cell cultures.

(c) *Understand the quality of the herbs*

All herbal formulae, once proven efficacious on a clinical problem would need to be further authenticated. One wants to get the best provision of the herb so that clinical effects could be guaranteed.

Basic records of quality control are established through chromatography studies (HPLC) while the species details related to origin of production are established with DNA finger printing.

Since quality suppliers of herbs are difficult to find, every item should have been subjected to counter-checks with standard extracts provided by the relevant academic institution in China (Standard Sample Extracts, 2003).

Stability tests, as required by registration authorities, need to be completed as routines.

(d) *Prepare for the improvement and optimisation of the formula*

Herbal formulae achieve additive and supplementary effects by mixing many herbs together. However, if the number of herbs is large, development by manipulating the formula becomes difficult. Four to five herbs in a formula might be the optimal number. When too many items are found in the classic formula, one could use modern concepts of pathology as guidelines to reduce the number. Since modern medicine works on direct targets, herbs advocated for direct actions could be considered for elimination because they are used together with modern medicine which already offers direct actions. Those herbs that are understood to be immuno-modulating and promoting anabolism will be kept. In other words, when the major action of a herb is already covered by modern medicine, the herb could be eliminated.

(e) *Rule out the possible interference with other pharmaceutical preparations being used*

Since mainstream clinical management is undoubtedly modern medicine, and TM-CAM preparation probably plays a supplementary role, it is important that the utilisation of the TM-CAM formula be tested against the modern medicine being used simultaneously, so as to prove that there are no adverse effects.

9.5 Conclusion and Recommendations

As the World Health Organization (WHO) advises that TM-CAM could be assessed in either one of the four ways, viz. evaluating in its own theoretical framework; in the theoretical framework of modern medicine; comparing its efficacy with modern medicine; and comparing with other systems of alternative medicine, one needs to decide, which way tends to be most fruitful (WHO, 2000).

I tend to believe that evaluating TM-CAM within the theoretical framework of modern medicine would be a way that is likely to give practical answers to difficult problems. This is a way that endorses modern scientific medicine as the mainstream management methodology of diseases and ailment, while at the same time trying to supplement deficiencies in the mainstream treatment. This is probably a way that is able to gain wide general acceptance. One method of implementing this evaluation could be achieved through the efficacy driven approach.

Recommendations

The recommendations on the line of approach for research on TM-CAM are summarised as follows:

(a) A specific clinical problem is identified by the clinician in a specific specialty. This problem is well known to all experts in the specialty and, in spite of past efforts, no satisfactory solution is yet available.
(b) Thorough literature search on TM-CAM is given to look for a possible solution. This includes classics in Chinese Medicine, recent reports and current literature.
(c) Consultation with TM-CAM experts: those who are involved with clinical work; and those who are herbal experts.
(d) Work out a practical option for the resolution of the clinical problem by creating a herbal formula (or other modality) for the treatment trial. This formula should preferably be a simple one that contains three to five herbs.
(e) Maintain a quality supply of herbal preparation for the clinical trial, bearing in mind:

(i) *Good Agricultural Practice* (*GAP*)

Watch out for slow materialisation of the GAP principles mainly from China. Before this becomes practical, find the best supplier.

(ii) Sufficient quantity should be bought from one supplier to make sure that the same batch of supply is used for clinical trials and parallel laboratory tests.

(iii) The supplier should be checked for procedures during cultivation (soil, watering, fertilisers, insecticides, etc.), harvest, packing, storage, sorting, cleaning, distribution, etc.

(iv) *Good Manufacturing Practice* (*GMP*)

Many laboratories have been screened and subsequently endorsed as being qualified for the supply of GMP. Herbal preparations are more specialised and are different from the production of other pharmaceutical products. However, before a different set of guidelines is prepared for herbal preparations as a separate entity, one has to be satisfied with GMP at large.

(v) *Good Laboratory Practice* (*GLP*)

More straightforward GLP guidelines are available and laboratories are scrutinised and labelled accordingly. Since herbal preparations have to be excluded from harmful contaminations like heavy metals, insecticides and biological agents, laboratories supplying the screening processes should be GLP qualified.

(f) Work out a clinical protocol built on Evidence-Based Medicine (EBM) and Good Clinical Practice (GCP). The design should follow high quality demands on clinical research, i.e. proper randomisation with double blinding, placebo control.

(g) EMB, GCP should have biostatisticians' input, Hospital Ethics Committee approval and a good system of adverse effects reporting.

(h) A series of laboratory experiments go parallel with the clinical trial, with two fundamental intensions:

(i) To understand the mode of action of the herbal preparation through Cell Cultures, Bioassays.

(ii) To authenticate the herbs being used, so that proper labeling and quality control of the herbal product could be maintained. Authentication includes chemical finger printing (HPLC) and DNA finger printing.

(i) Optimisation of herbal formula

The outcome of the properly conducted clinical trial would be able to show the practical effects of the herbal formula. When these observations are well supported by parallel laboratory investigations, one finds good justifications to further improve the formula, i.e. optimise it. Optimisation processes include the following:

(i) Use Chinese Medicine classical principles, to critically scrutinise the herbal formula. There might be room for modifications.
(ii) Use modern principles of pathology and clinical sciences to look for eliminations and/or addition of certain herbs.
(iii) Verify the results of the optimisation with the same laboratory models.
(iv) It might be considered necessary or advisable to repeat the clinical trial using the optimised formula, particularly when pharmaceutical developers want to support.
(v) Pharmacists and drug scientists would work out whole series of pharmacodynamics and pharmacokinetics in their enthusiasm to participate in the drug development.

(j) Within this whole process of herbal research, the difficulties in striving to reach a world level of scientific acceptance need to be understood and thoroughly explained to any reviewer. The difficulties have arisen out of the absence of perfect uniformity in literature and philosophic interpretation, herbal nomenclature, GAP, Suppliers, GMP, unknown active principles and social/cultural attitudes.

References

Ayurveda Medicine (2000) *Strategic Plan on the Promotion of Folk Medicine.* WHO Publication.

Cheng, Y.C. (2000) A personal perspective on bringing Chinese medicine into mainstream medicine in the 21st century. In: *2001 Traditional Chinese Medicine and National Products.* Era Resources Publisher, Hong Kong, pp. 27–35.

Cinatl, J., Morgenstern, B. and Bauer, G. (2003) Glycyrrhizin, an active component of Liquorice roots, and replication of SARS associated coronavirus. *Lancet* **361**(9374), 2045–2046.

De Smet, P. and Accy, P.F. (eds.) (1996) Drug interactions with herbal and other non-toxic remedies. In: *Mechanisms of Drug Interactions.* Springer-Verlag, Berlin.

Eisenberg, D.M. (1998) Unconventional medicine in the USA — prevalence, costs and patterns of use. *New Engl. J. Med.* **328**(4), 246–252.

Eisenberg, D.M. and Roger, D.B. (1998) Trends in alternative medicine in the USA 1990–1997. *JAMA* **280**(9), 1569–1575.

Goldbeck, W.S., Dorozynski, A. and Gunnar, L. (1996) Complementary medicine is booming worldwide. *BMJ* **313**(7050), 131–133.

Hannallah, D., Peterson B. and Lieberma, J.R. (2002) Gene therapy in orthopaedic surgery. *JBJS* **84**, 1046–1061.

Kaptchuk, T.J. and Eisenberg, D.M. (1998) The persuasive appeal of alternative medicine. *Annu. Int. Med.* **129**, 1061–1065.

Klemman, A. (1975) *Medicine in Chinese Cultures: Comparative Studies of Health Care in China and Other Countries.* US Department of Health, Education and Welfare, Washington DC.

Lai, S.L. *Clinical Trials of Traditional Chinese Materia Medica.* Guangdong People's Publishing House, Guangzhou, 2002.

Leung, P.C. and Wong, M.W.N. (2002) A critical analysis of professional and academic publications on Traditional Chinese Medicine in China. *Am. J. Chin. Med.* **30**(1), 177–181.

Lieberman, J.R., Daluiski, C.P. and Eihorn, T. (2002) Role of growth factors in the repair of bone biology and clinical applications. *Biol. Clin. Appl.* **84**, 1032–1044.

National Centre for Scientific Research (CNRS) (1999) *Report on the Successes of Development of Drugs from Botanical Plants.* Special Report CNRS, France.

Standard Sample Extracts from Common Chinese Medicine Herbs (2003). Catalogue list 2003.

Streitberge, K. and Kleinhenz, J. (1998) Introducing a placebo needle into acupuncture research. *Lancet* **352**(9125), 364–365.

Suen, T.Y., Wang, S.F. and Wang, K.L. (1998) *Adverse Effects of Drug Treatment.* Peoples' Health Press, Beijing.

Tang, J.L., Zhau, S.Y. and Ernst, E. (1999) Review of randomised controlled trials of Traditional Chinese Medicine. *BMJ* **319**, 160–161.

Valecha, N. and Tripath, K.D. (1997) Artemisinin: current status in malaria. *Indian J. Pharmacol.* **29**, 71–75.

Vincent, C. and Lewith, G. (1995) Placebo controls for acupuncture studies. *J. R. Soc. Med.* **88**, 192–202.

Yu, Z.K. and Boa, A.H. (2000) Different herbs bearing the same functional name. *Chin. Tradit. Herbal Drugs* **31**(3), 234–237 (in Chinese).

WHO (2000) *General Guidelines for Methodologies on Research and Evaluation of Traditional Medicine.* WHO, Geneva.

Chapter 10

Study of XS0601 on Preventing Restenosis after Coronary Interventional Treatment*

Ke-ji Chen, Hao Xu, Da-zhuo Shi & Xiao-chang Ma

Abstract

To evaluate the effect of XS0601(consisting of active parts from *Ligusticum chuanxiong* Hort. and *Paeonia lactiflora* Pall.) in preventing clinical and angiographic restenosis after percutaneous coronary intervention (PCI), and to explore the probable mechanism in a Porcine Coronary Injury Model. **Methods:** In a clinical study, 108 coronary heart disease patients with successful PCI were randomised into 55 cases in a control (routine treatment) group and 53 cases in a XS0601 (routine treatment combined with XS0601) group. The recurrence of angina, clinical end-point events, changing of blood-stasis syndrome score (BSSS) and coronary angiography within 6 months after coronary angioplasty or/and stenting were observed. Logistic multivariate regression analysis was applied to analyse the related factor of restenosis demonstrated by angiography. In an experimental study, an intimal hyperplasia model was established by oversized balloon injury at mid-region of the left anterior descending (LAD) coronary arteries of China minipigs, with which the mechanism of XS0601 was explored. Probucol was served as the Western medicine control. Morphometric and angiographic analysis of the injured arteries was performed 4 weeks after balloon dilation. **Results:** Follow-up angiography was performed in 42 patients including 18 cases in XS0601 group (restenosis was observed in 7 patients) and 24 cases in control group (restenosis was observed in 17 patients), there was significant difference between the occurrence of restenosis in XS0601 and that in the control group ($P < 0.05$). The occurrence of clinical end-point events (death, nonfatal target lesion myocardial infarction,

*National Ninth Five-Year Project (No. 96-906-06-01).

coronary artery bypass graft surgery, or repeat target-vessel angioplasty) in the XS0601 group (18.8%) were significantly lower than that in the control group (40%) ($P < 0.05$). The recurrent angina was observed in 13 cases in XS0601 group, and there was a significant difference when compared with 27 cases in the control group ($P < 0.05$). There was also remarkable significance for the difference of baseline and follow-up BSSS between groups ($P < 0.01$). Logistic multivariate stepwise regress analysis and multivariate regress analysis of the related factors with restenosis confirmed by coronary angiography showed that the baseline BSSS and the difference of baseline and follow-up BSSS were important influencing factors on the occurrence of restenosis after interventional treatment ($P < 0.05$). The experimental study showed that XS0601 can significantly reduce intimal thickness and pathological vascular remodeling 4 weeks after balloon injury ($P < 0.05$ or $P < 0.01$), thus reducing late lumen loss. **Conclusion:** In this pilot study, XS0601 can markedly reduce the occurrence of angiographic restenosis, clinical end-point events and recurrent angina, improve condition of blood-stasis after PCI. The severity of blood-stasis syndrome was an important influencing factor on the occurrence of restenosis. Inhibiting intimal thickness and pathological vascular remodeling may be the mechanism of XS0601 in preventing restenosis after PCI. It still needs to be further demonstrated by a large-scale, double-blinded, randomised and controlled study.

Keywords: XS0601; Angioplasty; Stent; Restenosis; Remodeling.

10.1 Introduction

Since percutaneous coronary intervention (PCI) can reconstruct coronary blood circulation without thoracotomy, it has become one of the main effective treatments for coronary heart disease. However, restenosis is a major limitation to the long-term success of this procedure. Despite numerous trials of pharmacological interventions, including anti-platelet agents, heparin, coronary vasodilators, ACEI, and fish oils, the frequency of restenosis has not diminished since the inception of PTCA. Coronary stents are the only devices that have shown a reduction in the incidence of restenosis, although it is still about 22%–29% (Hong *et al.*, 1997). The prevention of restenosis after PCI has become one of the major problems in the arena of cardiology.

The pathogenesis of restenosis is complex and not fully understood. According to the theory of Traditional Chinese Medicine (TCM), restenosis falls into the category of blood-stasis syndrome. Our previous studies (one of National Eighth Five-Year projects) have shown that Concentrated Xufu Zhuyu Pill (a classic formula of promoting blood circulation and removing blood-stasis) had a certain effect on preventing restenosis (Shi *et al.*, 1995; 1997). XS0601 consists of the main active position of *Ligusticum chuanxiong* Hort. and *Paeonia lactiflora* Pall. (both are the main ingredients in Concentrated Xufu Zhuyu Pill). In this study, we observe its clinical effect on preventing restenosis after PCI in patients with coronary heart disease (CHD), and to explore the probable mechanism in a porcine coronary injury model.

10.2 Methods

10.2.1 *Clinical study*

10.2.1.1 Diagnostic criteria

The diagnostic criteria of CHD refers to related criteria on ischemic heart disease of WHO (Chen, 1995). The diagnostic criteria of blood-stasis syndrome consults the criteria formulated by the Specialised Committee of Promoting Blood Circulation and Removing Blood-Stasis in China Society of Integrated Chinese and Western Medicine (CJIM, 1987). The symptoms and signs of blood stasis including angina, purple and dark tongue or with ecchymosis, purple and dark lip and gingiva, sublingual varices, uneven pulse or slow pulse with irregular intervals were scored according to methods introduced by literature (Wang, 1993). Since some patients in this study were suffering from acute myocardial infarction, the item of symptom (angina) was replenished "acute myocardial infarction" and the score was 15.

10.2.1.2 Patient selection and inclusion and exclusion criteria

Patients were enrolled between January 1999 and February 2000 in The Third Hospital Affiliated to Peking University and Anzhen Hospital Affiliated to Capital University of Medical Sciences. Patients were eligible for inclusion if they were 35 to 75 years old, had angina, and/or objective evidence of myocardial ischemia, or acute myocardial infarction, and there

Table 10.1. Baseline clinical and angiographic characteristics.

Variables	XS0601 group (n = 53)	Control group (n = 55)	P value
Demographics			
Age (yr)	55.3 ± 9.0	58.7 ± 9.12	> 0.05
Male	41 (77.4%)	46 (83.6%)	> 0.05
Smoking histroy	30 (56.6%)	34 (61.8%)	> 0.05
Systemic hypertension	28 (52.8%)	29 (52.7%)	> 0.05
Diabetes mellitus	7 (13.2%)	10 (18.2%)	> 0.05
Diagnosis			
UA	22 (41.5%)	28 (50.9%)	> 0.05
SA	8 (15.1%)	5 (9.1%)	> 0.05
AMI	22 (41.5%)	21 (38.2%)	> 0.05
Emergency treatment	5 (9.4%)	4 (7.3%)	> 0.05
No. of diseased vessels			
1	23 (43.4%)	19 (34.6%)	> 0.05
2	20 (37.7%)	23 (41.8%)	> 0.05
3	10 (18.9%)	13 (23.6%)	> 0.05
Lesion location	84	91	
LM	0	1 (1.1%)	> 0.05
LAD	44 (52.4%)	45 (49.5%)	> 0.05
LCx	28 (33.3%)	16 (17.6%)	> 0.05
RCA	12 (14.3%)	29 (31.9%)	> 0.05
Lesion classification (%)			
A	6 (7.14%)	7 (7.69%)	> 0.05
B1	36 (42.9%)	47 (51.7%)	> 0.05
B2	16 (19.1%)	15 (16.5%)	> 0.05
C	26 (31.0%)	22 (24.2%)	> 0.05
Stenting (lesion)	65 (77.4%)	69 (75.8%)	> 0.05
Stenosis > 85%	56 (66.7%)	59 (64.8%)	> 0.05

was at least one significant (> 50%) stenosis that was documented on a recent coronary angiogram, and with successful PTCA and/or coronary stenting. Patients were excluded if they met any of the following criteria: insulin-dependent diabetes, severe uncontrolled hypertension, severe renal or hepatic impairment, participation in another study. 108 enrolled patients were randomised into routine Western medicine treatment group (control group) and routine treatment plus XS0601 group (XS0601 group). The baseline characteristics of the patients are given in detail in Table 10.1. The groups were all matched for all variables ($P > 0.05$).

10.2.1.3 Treatment protocol

Standard balloon angioplasty was performed through the transfemoral approach according to standard techniques (Chen, 1994). After written informed consent was obtained, patients were randomised to receive routine treatment including aspirin, ticlopidine, heparin, calcium antagonists, etc. or routine treatment combined with XS0601 (consists of Chuanxingol and paeoniflorin and produced by the Chinese Medicine Institute of Suzhou Medical College; each capsule contains 0.25 g medicinal powder which corresponds to 7.5 g crude herbs, and was consumed 3 times a day and 0.5 g each time. Batch number: 980501), which begins from the day of interventional treatment until 6 months afterward. They were asked not to take additional Chinese medicine. Patient compliance with treatment was monitored by counting the returned bottles of XS0601. The clinical follow-up visit was scheduled 1 month after interventional treatment for determining whether there is recurrent angina and side-effects, and 6 months after treatment for follow-up angiography, treadmill exercise test, or myocardial nuclide imaging.

10.2.1.4 Clinical and angiographic end-points

The primary end-point was angiographic restenosis defined as a residual stenosis of < 50% after angioplasty that became ≥ 50% at follow-up. Clinical end-points were the occurrence of death, non-fatal target lesion myocardial infarction, coronary artery bypass graft surgery, or repeat target-vessel angioplasty within 6 months after the procedure.

10.2.2 *Experimental study*

10.2.2.1 Animals

We studied 24 Chinese minipigs weighing between 28 and 36 kg. The animals were randomised into four groups. Group 1 (control) consisted of seven untreated animals. Groups 2 to 4 received different drugs beginning 2 days before balloon injury and continuing throughout the 4-week study period. Group 2 (probucol) included six swine that received probucol 2000 mg once a day. Groups 3 and 4 (low-dose XS0601, LXS and high-dose XS0601, HXS) included six and five minipigs and received 0.02 g/kg and 0.04 g/kg, respectively. The drugs were crushed to powder form and mixed with corn syrup before being administered. The animals were observed to ensure the medication was taken. All animals were fed a normolipemic diet.

10.2.2.2 Experimental protocol

The experimental protocol referred to slightly modified methods introduced by Schneider *et al.* (1993). Twenty-four animals were pre-medicated with aspirin 325 mg and diltiazem HCl 60 mg the day before the procedure. The animals were sedated with a combination of ketamine (25 mg/kg) and diazepam (1 mg/kg), administered in combination by intramuscular injection. Overstretch-balloon injury was performed with a 20 mm-length PTCA catheter so that the inflated balloon-to-artery ratio was ≈ 1:4. It was advanced to the mid-segment of the LAD and three 30-second inflations were performed at 10 atm, and each inflation was separated by a 1-minute deflation period to allow for coronary perfusion. Uninstrumented LCx was used as a control. The animals were killed 4 weeks after the initial overstretch injury, the heart was rapidly excised through a left thoracotomy. The left main coronary artery was perfusion-fixed and serial 4 mm sections were then processed and embedded in paraffin. Cross-sections (4 μm thick) were stained with haematoxylin-eosin and Verhoeff-van Gieson stains. Angiography was performed in similar 45° left anterior oblique (LAO) view before, right after and 4 weeks after PTCA and recorded on videotape for analysis later.

Table 10.2. Histopathological grading system.

Grade	Criteria
0	No injury noted
1	IEL disrupted; media compressed not lacerated
2	IEL disrupted; medial visibly lacerated
3	EEL disrupted

10.2.2.3 Morphometric analysis

The presence of intimal proliferation, luminal encroachment, medial dissection, alteration of the internal elastic lamina (IEL) and external elastic lamina (EEL) were evaluated by an experienced cardiovascular pathologist blinded to the treatment group. A grading system based on the criteria (Schwartz *et al.*, 1992) listed in Table 10.2 was applied to the most reactive segment. Morphometric analysis was performed on the section of each artery with the largest neointimal lesion using a computerised colour image analysis system (Huizhong Company, China): the maximal intimal thickness (MIT, millimetres, determined by a line between the lumen and outermost point of the neointima), circumference of the IEL (IELc, millimetres) and its fracture length (IELf, millimetres). The extent of injury (injury score, IS) is represented by the IELf, standardised for the size of the artery, expressed by the IELc: IELf/IELc. Area measurements were obtained by tracing the lumen, IEL and EEL: lumen area (LA, square millimetres), area delimited by the IEL (IELa, square millimetres), area delimited by the EEL (EELa, square millimetres). Thus, media area (MA, square millimetres) could be obtained by subtracting IELa from EELa and intima area (IA, square millimetres) could be generated by subtracting lumen area from IELa. The residual lumen (RL) was expressed by lumen area/IELa. Proliferation index (PI) was expressed by IA/EELa. According to Bonan *et al.* (1993), restenosis injury index (RII) could provide a more accurate means of assessing the extent of restenostic response to a given injury and was expressed by PI/IS.

To quantitatively assessing the separate contributions of intimal hyperplasia and arterial remodeling to angiographic late lumen loss according to methods introduced by Post *et al.* (1994), we defined the following values: the potential cross-sectional lumen area was calculated from the perimeter of the IEL, assuming a circular configuration. The actual cross-sectional area was obtained by subtracting the area of intima from the potential lumen area. The difference between the radius of potential and actual lumen, as derived from their respective cross-sectional areas, was taken as the average thickness of neointima. Thus artery remodeling can be obtained by subtracting the doubled average thickness of neointima from late lumen loss. The late lumen loss can be obtained by the following angiographic analysis. The contribution of neointimal thickness or remodeling to late lumen loss could be calculated by dividing late lumen loss by neointimal thickness or remodeling.

10.2.2.4 Transmission electron microscopy

Tissue samples were fixed at 4°C in 2.5% glutaraldehyde, post-fixed in 1% osmium tetroxyde, dehydrated and embedded in Epon 812. The lesion (intima) was located by semi-thin section. The slice was prepared by ultrasection, stained with uranyl acetate and lead citrate and examined in a JEM-1200EX transmission electron microscope (Japan). The morphological criteria used for recognition of SMCs were the presence of basal lamina, plasmalemmal vesicles, and myofilament bundles with associated dense bodies. Only cell profiles of sufficient size to be characterised as SMCs by those criteria were analysed.

10.2.2.5 Angiographic analysis

Angiography analysis was performed on the cinefilms obtained during the baseline study (initial balloon injury) and follow-up study (when the animals were sacrificed). The measurements included the arterial diameters of the injury site before, after balloon dilations and at follow-up as well as the balloon-to-artery ratio. Thus the acute gain and late lumen loss can be obtained. The minimum angiographic lumen diameter was measured by an angiographer blinded to treatment groups. For the arterial diameters, they were corrected for angiographic magnification. The magnification factor was determined by dividing the angiographic balloon diameter by the *ex vivo*-measured balloon diameter.

10.2.3 *Statistical analysis*

The statistical analysis was performed with STATA 4.0 software. All tests were two-tailed, and values of $P < 0.05$ were considered significant. T test was used for comparison of quantitative data and X^2 test was used for enumeration data. For related factors of angiographic restenosis, logistic multivariate stepwise regress analysis and logistic multivariate regress analysis were applied. To determine whether there were any difference between the groups in the timing of clinical events, the data were also analysed using the Kaplan-Meier model.

10.3 Results

10.3.1 *Clinical study*

10.3.1.1 Comparison of recurrent angina

Clinical follow-up was available for all patients after 6 months. During the 6th-month follow-up, recurrent angina was seen in 13 cases in the XS0601 group (no AMI), while 27 cases were seen in the control group (six patients were diagnosed with AMI). There was significant difference between the XS0601 and the control groups ($P < 0.05$). See Table 10.3.

10.3.1.2 Angiographic analysis

Angiographic follow-up was obtained in 42 patients (67 lesions) 166.62 ± 67.62 days after interventional treatment. The angiographic follow-up rate was 38.89%. The mean angiographic follow-up time was 168.71 ± 58.93 days and 165.15 ± 74.57 days after treatment, respectively ($P > 0.05$).

Table 10.3. Recurrent angina between groups.

	n	Without angina	Angina
XS0601 group	53	40 (75.5%)	13 (24.5%)*
Control group	55	28 (50.9%)	27 (49.1%)

Note: Compared with control group, *$P < 0.05$.

The primary end-point of restenosis defined as ≥ 50% diameter stenosis at follow-up occurred in seven of 18 patients in XS0601 group (new lesions occurred in the other two cases without restenosis) and in 17 of 24 patients in the control group (among whom new lesions occurred in six cases), there was significant difference between groups ($P < 0.05$). Similarly, restenosis occurred in seven of 22 lesions in the XS0601 group and in 25 of 45 lesions in the control group, although there was no significant difference ($P = 0.092$). See Table 10.4.

10.3.1.3 Comparison of clinical events

Clinical follow-up was available for all patients. The incidence of clinical events (including death, non-fatal target lesion myocardial infarction, coronary artery bypass graft surgery, or repeat target-vessel angioplasty) during clinical follow-up in the two groups is shown in Table 10.5. The occurrence of clinical events in the XS0601 group (18.8%) was significantly lower than that in the control group (40%) ($P < 0.05$). See Fig. 10.1.

Table 10.4. Angiographic analysis between groups.

	Patients (42)		Lesions (67)	
	No restenosis	Restenosis	No restenosis	Restenosis
XS0601 group	11	7*	15	7
Control group	7	17	20	25

Note: Compared with control group, *$P < 0.05$.

Table 10.5. Comparison of clinical events.

	n	Death	AMI	Repeat PTCA	CABG	Total
XS0601 group	53	0	0	9	1	10 (18.87%)*
Control group	55	0	6	15	1	22 (40%)

Note: Compared with control group, *$P < 0.05$.

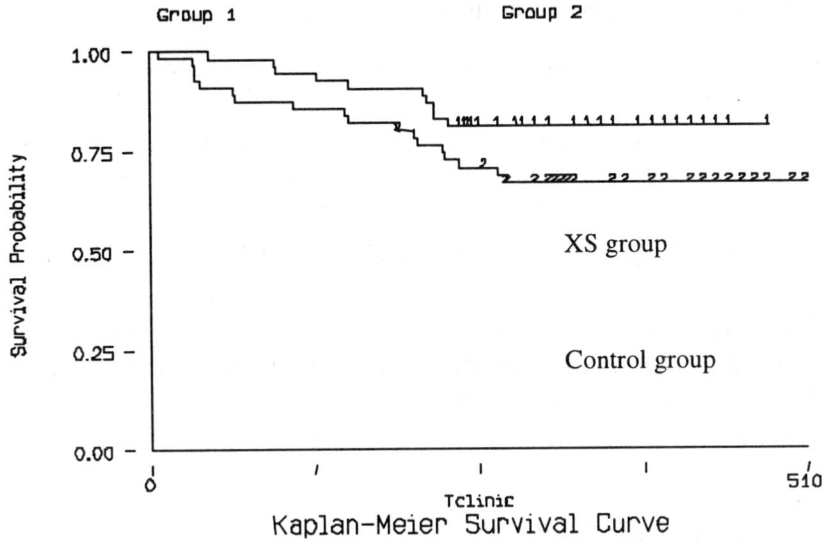

Figure 10.1. Comparison of event-free survival.

Table 10.6. Comparison of BSSS between groups.

		BSSS		
	n	Baseline	Follow-up	Difference
XS0601 group	53	22.74 ± 8.88	9.40 ± 8.08* △	13.34 ± 7.31*
Control group	55	21.96 ± 8.09	14.55 ± 9.38 △	7.42 ± 6.30

Note: Compared with control group, *P < 0.01; compared with baseline score, △P < 0.01.

10.3.1.4 Comparison of BSSS between groups

The baseline BSSS is similar between groups (P > 0.05). At 6 months after interventional treatment, BSSS was reduced significantly in both the XS0601 and the control groups as compared with the corresponding baseline values (P < 0.01). There was also significant difference of BSSS at 6th month follow-up and the BSSS difference between the XS0601 and the control groups (P < 0.01). See Table 10.6.

10.3.1.5 Logistic regression analysis

Logistic multivariate stepwise regression analysis was used to identify predictors (a total of 27 factors including age, sex, hypertension, diabetes, history of smoking, family history, diagnosis, pre-MI, recurrent angina, type of TCM syndrome, baseline BSSS, BSSS at follow-up, the difference of baseline BSSS and BSSS at follow-up, number of arteries involved, WBC, RBC, PLT, HCT, TC, TG, HDL, LDL, TC/HDL, blood sugar, treatment with ACEI, treatment with HMG-CoA reductase inhibitors, and treatment with XS0601) of patients with restenosis demonstrated by angiography. The results showed that baseline BSSS and the difference of baseline and follow-up BSSS were important influencing factors on the occurrence of restenosis after interventional treatment ($P < 0.05$).

10.3.2 *Experimental study*

Group characteristics are listed in Table 10.7. There were no significant differences in animal weight at the time of balloon injury. Of the 24 animals, four died within 24 hours of the procedure. The causes of death included ventricular fibrillation ($n = 3$, one each in the control, probucol and LXS groups) and delayed acute myocardial infarction associated with thrombosis ($n = 1$, in the control group). There was no evidence that any of the drugs used contributed to the deaths. Excluding those animals that did not survive the procedure, rupture of IEL was seen in all animals. There were five pigs in each group for the final analysis. The angiographic balloon-to-artery ratio and dilation after injury, the pathological grade and injury score based on analysis of histopathology were similar among groups.

10.3.2.1 Histopathological analysis

To document coronary artery injury and characterise the neointima, histopathological analysis of all artery segments was performed. As shown in Fig. 10.2, there was rupture of the IEL with neointimal growth replacing the disrupted media at 4 weeks after injury. The neointima consisted of smooth muscle cells (SMCs), loose connective tissue, and proteoglycans,

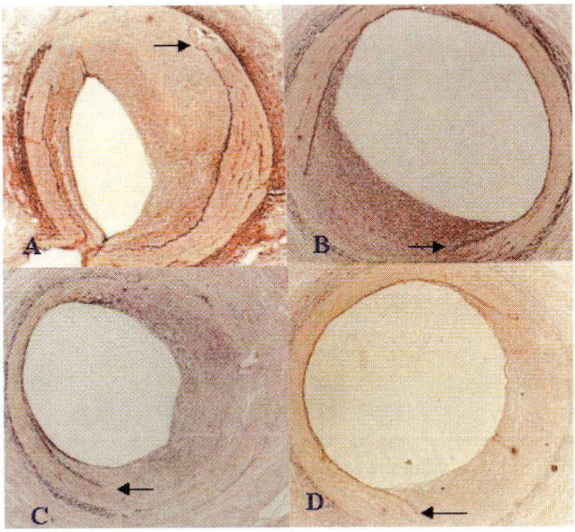

Figure 10.2. Representative histological cross-sections of coronary arteries 4 weeks after balloon injury (Verhoeff-van Gieson elastin stain, × 50). A: Control group, B: probucol group, C: low-dose XS0601 group, and D: high-dose XS0601 group. Note similar disruption of the internal elastic lamina (⟶) at the site of intimal reaction in all groups and significant reduction of intimal hyperplasia in groups treated with different drugs, especially in the high-dose XS0601 group, compared with the control group.

as identified by light microscopy. Analysis of electron microscopy demonstrated that the dominant cell type in neointima was SMCs. Besides, there were also a small number of fibroblasts and rare macrophages. Injury (rupture of IEL) was documented in all animals with similar histopathological grade between groups (Table 10.7).

10.3.2.2 Morphometric analysis

General comparison between the treatment and control groups including MIT, injury score, LA, IELa, EELa, MA, IA, RL (%), PI and RII are listed in Tables 10.7 and 10.8. HXS could significantly reduce MIT (0.34 ± 0.05) and RII (0.37 ± 0.07) compared with the control group (0.89 ± 0.40 and 1.14 ± 0.51, respectively) ($P < 0.05$). Since intimal hyperplasia after balloon dilation varied in proportion to injury in this model, quantitative

Table 10.7. Baseline, angiographic and histopathological characteristics.

Characteristics	Control	Probucol	LXS	HXS
Minipig	7	6	6	5
No. of death(s)	2	1	1	0
Weight (kg)	32.4 ± 3.36	31 ± 2.74	32 ± 3.32	30.4 ± 2.19
Angiography				
Balloon-to-artery ratio	1.40 ± 0.04	1.37 ± 0.10	1.37 ± 0.09	1.42 ± 0.06
Dilation (after injury)(%)	21.21 ± 0.06	22.24 ± 0.09	24.99 ± 0.09	23.69 ± 0.05
Histopathology				
Pathological grade	2.6 ± 0.89	2.6 ± 0.89	3 ± 0	2.4 ± 0.89
Injury score	0.35 ± 0.18	0.31 ± 0.20	0.31 ± 0.11	0.41 ± 0.20

Values are mean ± SD. No values were significantly different among the four groups by ANOVA ($P > 0.05$).

Table 10.8. Morphometric analysis.

	Control	Probucol	LXS	HXS
MIT (mm)	0.89 ± 0.40	0.54 ± 0.15	0.48 ± 0.08	0.34 ± 0.05*
LA (mm^2)	0.90 ± 1.18	1.35 ± 0.83	1.88 ± 0.91	2.01 ± 0.88†
IELa (mm^2)	2.20 ± 0.65	2.16 ± 0.64	2.62 ± 1.03	2.52 ± 0.76
EELa (mm^2)	3.22 ± 0.63	3.34 ± 0.62	3.68 ± 1.18	3.40 ± 0.64
MA (mm^2)	1.02 ± 0.11	1.18 ± 0.43	1.06 ± 0.47	0.88 ± 0.30
IA (mm^2)	1.30 ± 0.68	0.81 ± 0.68	0.74 ± 0.14	0.51 ± 0.27
RL (%)	34 ± 37	62 ± 24*	70 ± 7†	77 ± 14†
PI	0.43 ± 0.23	0.24 ± 0.18*	0.21 ± 0.04†	0.16 ± 0.09†
RII	1.14 ± 0.51	0.69 ± 0.26	0.72 ± 0.14	0.37 ± 0.07*

Values are mean ± SD. *$P < 0.05$, significance *versus* control: comparison of group means after ANOVA; *$P < 0.05$, †$P < 0.01$, significance *versus* control: comparison of group means after ANOVA taking injury score as covariance.

group comparisons were performed in which the vessel injury score was used as a covariance. After essential test of mutual effect (injury score and group) and linear relationship (with injury score), covariance analysis was applied to LA, RL and PI. Both probucol and XS could markedly raise RL and decrease PI compared with the control group ($P < 0.05$),

(P < 0.01). HXS could also increase LA at four weeks after injury compared with the control group (P < 0.05).

10.3.2.3 Angiographic analysis

Angiographic analysis was performed by digital calipers to determine the arterial diameter before and after balloon injury, the balloon-to-artery ratio, and the arterial diameter at the time of follow-up. Thus acute gain, dilation, late loss of lumen could be obtained. As presented in Tables 10.7, 10.9 and 10.10, the arterial diameter before and after balloon injury, the balloon-to-artery ratio, dilation and acute gain were similar between groups. All of the drug groups seemed to lower late lumen loss and increase the arterial diameter at the time of follow-up compared to the control group, but there was no significant difference among groups (P > 0.05). Taking acute gain as covariances, both XS0601 and probucol could markedly reduce angiographic late lumen loss and late lumen loss resulting from intimal hyperplasia (P < 0.05, P < 0.01), which is similar to the morphometric analysis. LXS and HXS could also significantly increase the arterial diameter at the time of follow-up and reduce late lumen loss resulting from remodeling (P < 0.05, P < 0.01).

Table 10.9. Angiographic analysis.

	Control	Probucol	LXS	HXS
Diameter (before, mm)	2.20 ± 0.33	2.05 ± 0.33	2.22 ± 0.49	2.12 ± 0.34
Diameter (after, mm)	2.66 ± 0.34	2.49 ± 0.30	2.75 ± 0.47	2.62 ± 0.45
Diameter (follow-up, mm)	1.34 ± 0.82	1.75 ± 0.47	1.97 ± 0.51*	2.03 ± 0.30*
Acute gain (mm)	0.43 ± 0.17	0.51 ± 0.10	0.58 ± 0.03	0.55 ± 0.11
Late loss (mm)	1.32 ± 0.71	0.74 ± 0.39†	0.78 ± 0.33†	0.59 ± 0.28†

Values are mean ± SD. No values were significantly different between groups by ANOVA (P > 0.05).

*P < 0.05, †P < 0.01, significance *versus* control: comparison of group means after ANOVA taking acute gain as covariance.

Table 10.10. Effect of intimal thickness or remodeling on late lumen loss.

	Control	Probucol	LXS	HXS	
Combined late loss (mm)	1.32 ± 0.71	0.74 ± 0.39†	0.78 ± 0.33†	0.59 ± 0.28†	
Mean intimal thickness × 2 (mm)	0.71 ± 0.42	0.35 ± 0.29*	0.28 ± 0.03†	0.21 ± 0.12†	
Discrepancy (remodeling)	0.60 ± 0.39	0.39 ± 0.22	0.50 ± 0.31*	0.37 ± 0.23†	
Contribution of thickness (%)	51 ± 15	42 ± 19	44 ± 27	35 ± 19	41 ± 20
Contribution of remodeling (%)	49 ± 15	58 ± 19	56 ± 27	65 ± 19	59 ± 20

Values are mean ± SD. No values were significantly different between groups by ANOVA (P > 0.05).
*P < 0.05, †P < 0.01, significance *versus* control: comparison of group means after ANOVA taking acute gain as covariance.

10.3.2.4 Relationships between acute gain, late lumen loss, intimal area and remodeling

For all groups, late loss correlated significantly with acute gain: $r = 0.59$, $P < 0.01$, regression: late loss = (2.37 × acute gain) – 0.26. No correlation between acute gain and intimal area was observed $r = 0.39$, $P > 0.05$). The correlation between remodeling and acute gain was $r = 0.74$, $P < 0.01$, regression: remodeling = (1.63 × acute gain) – 0.30. There was also correlation between remodeling and intimal area: $r = 0.51$, $P < 0.01$, regression: remodeling = (0.25 × intimal area) + 0.25.

10.3.2.5 Contribution of intimal hyperplasia and remodeling to late loss

The contribution of intimal thickness or remodeling to late lumen loss was similar among groups ($P > 0.05$). To sum up the results in the four groups, the percentage of late loss explained by intimal thickness was 41 ± 20%, while remodeling accounted for 59 ± 20% of the observed angiographic late loss in lumen diameter. See Table 10.5.

10.4 Discussion

The pathogenesis of restenosis is complex and not fully understood. However, it is well accepted that the main initial factor of restenosis is adhesion and aggregation of platelets resulting from vascular injury by balloon dilation, which leads to secretion of some chemokines and mitogens such as platelet-derived growth factor (PDGF) and basic fibroblast growth factor (bFGF). These growth factors promote abnormal expression of proto-oncogens and synthesis of protein for regulating cell cycle, which initiate the course of restenosis including thrombosis, inflammation of vascular wall, proliferation of smooth muscle cell and accumulation of extracellular matrix (Hong *et al.*, 1997). This pathologic course is similar to "obstruction of heart vessel" in the theory of Traditional Chinese Medicine (TCM) and it belongs to the category of blood-stasis syndrome. Our previous studies (one of the Eighth Five-Year projects) have shown that there is a certain relationship between restenosis and blood-stasis, and Concentrated Xufu Zhuyu Pill (a classic formula of promoting blood circulation and removing blood-stasis) had certain effect on preventing restenosis and improving the condition of blood-stasis in patients (Shi *et al.*, 1997). Similar results were seen in another clinical study on 84 patients with coronary heart disease who received successful coronary stenting, although there was no significant difference on angiographic restenosis as compared with the control group due to the small sample size (Yu *et al.*, 1998).

Based on these studies, we simplified the prescription and chose *Ligusticum chuanxiong* Hort. and *Paeonia lactiflora* Pall. as the representative medicines in the above prescriptions, explored the optimum dosage proportion by orthogonal experimental design, extracted the main active position and made XS0601. The present clinical study showed that XS0601 could reduce occurrence of angiographic restenosis and clinical end-point events, reduce recurrent angina, as well as lower BSSS. The above results indicated that it could really improve the condition of blood-stasis in patients and prevent restenosis by the method of promoting blood circulation and removing blood-stasis, which further optimises prescription. By logistic regress analysis, the present study showed that the severity of blood-stasis syndrome was an important influencing factor on the occurrence of restenosis after interventional treatment. It not only provides the occurrence of restenosis with one of the predicting factors, but also provides intervening restenosis by the method of promoting blood circulation and removing blood-stasis with theoretical basis.

Recently, analysis from study results from different arteries, interventions, species and experimental conditions (Post *et al.*, 1994 and 1997) has consistently shown that intimal hyperplasia accounts for only a minor proportion of the observed angiographic late loss in lumen diameter. Vascular remodeling, defined as a structural change in total arterial circumference during the restenosis period, is recognised as a major component of the restenosis process (Di Mario *et al.*, 1995). In this angiographic and histological study of Chinese minipigs fed with a normolipemic diet, remodeling explained 59% of late lumen loss, and 41% explained intimal hyperplasia. Both intimal hyperplasia and vascular remodeling are important to late lumen loss in this porcine coronary injury model. XS0601 and probucol could markedly inhibit hyperplasia-related indexes obtained from morphometric analysis and reduce angiographic late lumen loss. XS0601 could also significantly reduce angiographic late lumen loss resulting from vascular remodeling. While there is no significant difference in the probucol group compared with the control group, a clear trend was noted. This study suggests that XS0601 could reduce both intimal hyperplasia and vascular remodeling in swine coronary artery after balloon injury and it might be one of the mechanisms of XS0601 in preventing restenosis after PCI.

During clinical follow-up after PTCA and/or coronary stenting, repeat angiography was still the most reliable index to determine the occurrence of restenosis. However, due to special conditions of China, most patients are reluctant to accept repeat angiography except for occurrence of typical angina. The repeat angiographic rate in China is only about 10%–30%. Although the angiographic follow-up rate in this study is 38.89%, it is relatively low as compared with some large-scale clinical trials for preventing restenosis in foreign countries. Due to the limitation of present conditions, the sample size of this study was also small. On the basis of preliminary demonstration of XS0601 on preventing restenosis, a multi-center, large-scale, randomised, double-blinded and placebo-controlled clinical trial is essential.

Acknowledgements

The authors are indebted to Prof. Chen Mingzhe and Mao Jiemin of The Third Hospital, which is affiliated to Peiking University, and Prof. Lu Suzhen of Anzhen Hospital which is affiliated to the Capital University of Medical Sciences for their close coorperation on clinical research.

References

Bonan, R., Paiement, P., Scortichini, D., Cloutier, M.J. and Leung, T.K. (1993) Coronary restenosis: evaluation of a restenosis injury index in a swine model. *Am. Heart J.* **126**, 1334–1340.

Chen, H.Z. (1995) *Internal Medicine*, 1st Ed. The Peoples Medical Publishing House.

Chen, Z.J. (1994) *Clinical Coronary Heart Disease*, 1st Ed. Publishing House of People Military Surgeon.

Di Mario, C., Gil, R., Camenzind, E., Ozaki, Y,, Von Birgelen, C., Umans, V., De Jaegere, P., de Feyter, P.J., Roelandt, J.R. and Surruys, P.W. (1995) Quantitative assessment with intracoronary ultrasound of the mechanisms of restenosis after percutaneous transluminal coronary angioplasty and directional coronary atherectomy. *Am. J. Cardiol.* **75**, 772–777.

Hong, M.K., Mehran, R., Mintz, G.S., *et al.* (1997) Restenosis after coronary angioplasty. *Curr. Probl. Cardiol.* **22**(1), 7–36.

Post, M.J., Borst, C. and Kuntz, R.E. (1994) The relative importance of arterial remodeling compared with intimal hyperplasia in lumen renarrowing after balloon angioplasty: a study in the normal rabbit and the hypercholesterolemic Yucatan micropig. *Circulation* **89**, 2816–2821.

Post, M.J., de Smet, B.J., Helm, Y., Borst, C. and Kuntz, R.E. (1997) Arterial remodeling after balloon angioplasty or stenting in an atherosclerotic experimental model. *Circulation* **96**, 996–1003.

Schneider, J.E., Berk, B.C., Gravanis, M.B., *et al.* (1993) Probucol decrease neointimal formation in a swine model of coronary artery balloon injury: a possible role for antioxidants in restenosis. *Circulation* **88**, 628–637.

Schwartz, R.S., Huber, K.C., Murphy, J.G., Edwards, W.D., Camrud, A.R., Vlietstra, R.E. and Holmes, D.R. (1992). Restenosis and the proportional neointimal response to coronary artery injury: results in a porcine model. *J. Am. Coll. Cardiol.* **19**, 267–274.

Shi, D.Z., Li, J., Ma, X.C., *et al.* (1997) Clinical observation of concentrated Xufu Zhuyu Pill on preventing restenosis after percutaneous transluminal coronary angioplasty in patients of coronary heart disease. *Chin. J. Tradit. Chin. Med.* **38**(1), 27–29.

Shi, D.Z., Xu, F.Q., Ma, X.C., *et al.* (1995) The experimental study of Xuc Guan Tong on preventing restenosis after percutaneous transluminal angioplasty. *CJIW* **1**(4), 284–287.

The Specialty Committee of Promoting Blood Circulation and Removing Blood-stasis of China Association of Integrative Western and Chinese Medicine (1987) The diagnostic criteria of blood-stasis syndrome. *CJIM* **7**(3), 129.

Wang, J. (1993) *Study on Diagnostic Criteria of Blood-Stasis Syndrome. Research and Clinical Application of Promoting Blood Circulation and Removing Blood-stasis,* 1st Ed. The United Publishing House of Beijing Medical University and China Union Medical University.

Yu, B., Chen, K.J. and Mao, J.M. (1998) Clinical study of concentrated Xufu Zhuyu Pill on preventing restenosis after coronary stenting in patients of coronary heart disease. *CJIM* **18**(10), 585–589.

Chapter 11

Research on Treatment of AIDS in Chinese Medicine

Chong-fen Guan

Abstract

Despite the advances in the modern treatment of AIDS which include new drugs and different forms of combined therapy on "cocktails", the treatment of the disease is far from satisfactory. Drug toxicities and the readiness to develop drug resistance are major obstacles to the control of this devastating disease. It would be a real blessing if traditional/alternative medicine could be used to fight AIDS.

Although no conclusion could yet be drawn on the effectiveness of Chinese herbs against AIDS, a number of interesting clinical observations and laboratory studies have demonstrated the possibility of efficacy. Studies were centered around the immuno-modulating effects of some herbs and herbal formulae. Explorations are being done on the anti-viral effects of some other herbs and herbal formulae.

It is the author's opinion that future studies should follow international diagnostic standards and criteria of evaluation.

Keywords: Chinese Medicine; AIDS; Herbal Therapy.

11.1 Introduction

In 1981, the United States reported the first case of AIDS. Today, the number of global HIV-infected patients is over 40 million, and nearly half of them have died. The number of AIDS infection in China is estimated to be over 800,000. Thus, there is an urgent need to take the preventive and treatment measures. To implement the "prevention first" principle, pharmaceutical therapy would also be an important measure to control the development of pandemic situation.

Traditional Chinese Medicine (TCM) has several thousand years history in the prevention and treatment of diseases. It has a complete theoretical system and abundant clinical experience, which has contributed greatly to the health of mankind. AIDS is a new disease, with only a history of ten-odd years. The main theory of traditional Chinese medicine is to treat diseases with differentiation of syndromes, stressing the holistic and dynamic perspective. Experts of traditional Chinese medicine have made a lot of progress in the treatment and prevention of AIDS through their clinical and experimental researches. More studies are expected to make further contributions to combat this fatal disease (Lu *et al.*, 2002).

11.2 Clinical Research of Treating AIDS by CM

Based on the basic syndrome differentiation theory of CM, after clinical pattern classification and by applying the treating principle, the cases are treated with the prescriptions composed of Chinese medicine. In some areas of the world, a lot of work has been done and some progress has been made.

Chen (1989) treated AIDS cases in three stages. In the first stage, fornoxious dampness, the principle of removing pathogenic heat from blood, eliminating pathogenic heat from the blood is adopted, and "Gan Lu Xiao Du Yin" is prescribed. In the second stage, the principle of invigorating primordial energy is adopted, and the prescription "Sheng Mai Yin" is used. In the third stage, the principle of strengthening the body resistance and restoring the normal functions of the body to consolidate the constitution and tonify both *qi* and blood is adopted, with the prescription "Gui Pi Tang", which aims at relieving symptoms and prolonging life span.

Su (1992) analysed 30 cases of AIDS treated with TCM in collaboration with Tanzania. The cases were divided into four patterns, i.e. (1) deficiency of Yin fluid of both the lung and the kidney systems, (2) weakness of the spleen and the stomach systems, (3) deficiency of both the spleen and the kidney systems, and (4) excessive heat and phlegm accumulation pattern. After treatment with the principle of differentiation of syndromes, both symptoms and clinical examination data of patients were improved.

Huang (1990) classified AIDS cases into body weakness and exopathy pattern, and chronic debility pattern. The following therapeutic methods were adopted: enhancing the immunity of the body, where Radix Ginseng, Radix Astragali, etc. were used; for anti-infection, where Flos Lonicerae, Herba Taraxaci, folium Isatidis, etc. were used.

Zhao (1989) suggested that, in the early stage, the cases can be treated with "Huang Qi Sheng Mai Yin" and "Gui Pi Tang"; in relevant comprehensive stage, the cases can be treated with "Shen Ling Bai Shu Wan" and "Liu Jun Zi Tang".

Li (1994a) held that, as AIDS is caused by viral infection, it is pertaining to "epidemic disease" in TCM. In clinical treatment, it may be divided into five patterns, i.e. Yin and Yang deficiency in the lung system; deficiency of both the lung and spleen systems; deficiency of both *qi* and Yin in heart system; deficiency of both the spleen and the kidney systems; and noxious heat and heat-phlegm pattern.

Wang *et al.* (1995) held that, in the treatment of AIDS, no symptoms are to be differentiated in the early stage (AC stage). Only differentiation of diseases can be performed. A fixed prescription composing drugs with the effects of expelling evil factors (anti-HIV) and strengthening the body resistance (enhancing immunity) may be used. In the intermediate or late stage (ARC, AIDS), due to the occurrence of accidental infections and tumour, more complicated conditions, impairments of various organs caused by various pathogens, differentiation of syndromes is a priority in treatment. A definite formula will be prescribed accordingly.

The Yun Nan Institute of Traditional Chinese Medicine treated 37 cases of HIV infection caused by venous drug-injection with "Qian Kun Ning". After treatment, the patients with CD4 increased $> 40/mm^3$ amounted to 11 cases. The body weight of the patients increased 4.15 kg in average. The symptoms of lassitude, night sweat and cough were relieved (Li, 1995).

Li *et al.* (1996) have achieved good results in the treatment of 27 cases of AIDS with their self-made Chinese medicine "Sheng Ming Quan".

Fu *et al.* (1994) treated three cases of AIDS. A six-year follow-up study showed that their conditions were stable, their immunological functions were basically normal, and their symptoms improved.

Yoichi (1988) reported treatment of seven cases of AIDS with glycyrrhizin. As a result, an increase of CD4/CD8 value was seen in seven cases and an increase of CD4 cell number in four cases.

In Japan, 13 institutes jointly treated 56 cases of HIV infection with Xiao Chai Hu Tang and Ren Shen Tang. The results indicate the effectiveness of this remedy in improving the immunological function of the HIV carriers and increasing their body weight (Masao, 1988).

Goh *et al.* (1994) reported 130 cases of AIDS treated with "Medicinal Tea No. 1". The results indicated a decrease of opportunistic infection, an increase of body weight, and a marked elevation of number of CD4 cell, CD4/CD8 value and number of red blood cells.

Koji *et al.* (1994) reported the treatment of 40 cases of HIV-infected homosexuals with Chinese medicine Xiao Chai Hu Tang. The effective rate was 65%.

Krishnamurthy *et al.* (1995) treated 25 cases of HIV infection with Siddha Medicine-India-H-43 which consists of 43 kinds of medicinal plants. It was found that it can relieve symptoms, increase body weight, alleviate diarrhea, and restore working ability in most patients.

Alaka *et al.* (1995) reported on treatment of HIV infection with traditional herbal medicine. The effect was identical with that of AZT.

Since 1987, the China Academy of Traditional Chinese Medicine has dispatched TCM experts to Tanzania. In collaboration with local experts, they have treated around 10,000 cases of HIV/AIDS with TCM therapy, and carried out clinical observations in accordance with international diagnostic standards. One hundred and fifty-eight cases were treated with series of Chinese medicine, and a three-year observation indicated an effective rate of 39.87% (Lu *et al.*, 1992). Subsequently, 437 confirmed cases of AIDS were treated with Zhongyan Nos. 1 to 3 and a compound prescription of TCM Glyke. Four TCM types of clinical presentation were differentiated: (1) Lung-Stomach Yin Deficiency Type: early and middle-stage patients with the symptoms of respiratory system; (2) Spleen-Stomach Asthenia Type: middle stage patients with the symptoms of digestive system; (3) Spleen-Kidney Deficiency Type: mainly advanced stage patients; and (4) Excessive Heat with Confusion caused by Phlegm Type: terminal stage patients with involvement of central nervous system. Observations were made for three years. The results showed that symptoms were improved to a certain extent: body weight increased, and symptoms such as fatigue, diarrhea, cough, skin rash and lymphadenopathy were alleviated. The results of immunological function tests showed that two-thirds of the patients had an increased or stable CD4 cell number and CD4/CD8 value (60.32%). In addition, no side-effects of the herbal medicine were found in our research work, and the expense of the herbal medicine was lower than that of the western medicine (HARRT).

In our research, 32 HIV/AIDS patients from China and Tanzania, whose diagnosis comformed with the same standard, were observed clinically for three months after being administered with Chinese medicine Zhongyan No. 2 (ZY-2). The therapeutic effect was evaluated in terms of immune function viral load and clinical symptoms and signs. The results indicated that all of them could improve symptoms and enhance immune function, and CD4 count increased about 30% compared to those before treatment, of which 16 cases in Tanzania were carried out for viral load (VL), which was reduced over 0.5 log in seven cases. For the other 16 cases in China, the viral load was reduced in four cases. The total effective rate of clinical observation was about 47% (Guan *et al.*, 2003b).

Attempts were made to probe into the cases that were accompanied by opportunistic infection. Wu (1991a) treated AIDS accompanied by diarrhea with the principle of taking into account both Zheng (healthy energy) and Xie (evil forces), as well as Xu (deficiency) and Shi (excess), and achieved good results. Wang *et al.* (1994) reported that they had treated AIDS patients who had dark purple ecchymosis on tongue proper, pertaining to stagnation caused by deficiency of vital energy, with Chinese drugs that activate blood circulation and remove stasis and had achieved regulatory effects. In conclusion, the above-mentioned clinical practices suggested that treatment of AIDS with TCM therapy has achieved significant results, and thus warrants further research and wide application.

11.3 Experimental Research on CM for Anti-AIDS

11.3.1 *Screening of anti-HIV drugs*

(1) *Screening of single Chinese drugs and studies on their pharmacological function*

At the China Academy of Traditional Chinese Medicine, Guan (1993) screened *in vitro* more than 40 kinds of Chinese drugs for effective treatment of AIDS with SIV and HUT-78 cell line and discovered that inhibitory rates of Radix Glycyrrhizae, Herba Violae and Radix Trichosanthis on SIV positive cells were greater than 50%, and that of Radix Bupleuri, Indigo Naturalis and Flos Lonicerae were greater than 30%. Tan *et al.* (1992) screened more than 30 kinds of Chinese drugs with HIV-RT as target enzyme and discovered that the inhibitory rates of extracts of Ramulus Taxilli, Spica Prunellae, etc. on HIV-RT were above 30% when their concentration was 100 μg/ml. Luo *et al.* (1996) screened 700 commonly used Chinese drugs and selected 90 (13%) which had inhibitory effects on the AIDS virus. The selected drugs include Cortix Mori, Radix Arnebiae, Fructus Crotonis, etc. Jin *et al.* (1993) observed 14 kinds of Chinese drugs with HIV-infected MOLT-4 cell line *in vitro*. Among them, Radix Salviae Miltiorrhizae, Radix Bupleuri and Glycyrrhizin have better inhibitory effects on formation of fusion cell. Chang *et al.* (1988) screened 27 kinds of Chinese drugs which have the effect of clearing away heat and toxic materials with infected H9 cell line, and discovered that 11 of them (including Spica Prunellae, Herba Andrographitis, Fructus Arctii, Griseband Randix and Sophorae Flavescentis) have an inhibitory effect on HIV. Khansari and Mohraz (1995) extracted purified PPE from traditional medicinal plants with anti-virus activity which had 100% anti-HIV and anti-HTLV-I activities.

A large amount of work has been done in the field of pharmacological study of extracts of single Chinese drugs. Glycyrrhizin (GL) in Radix Glycyrrhizae can inhibit HIV antigen expression, formation of megalocaryocyte and HIV replication (Yamamoto, 1989). The extract of Radix Trichosanthis GLQ-223 can inhibit the activity of reverse transcriptase, prevent the release of P24 antigen and selectively kill the HIV-infected macrophage (Zhang, 1990). Baicalin and Baicalein extracted from

Radix Astragalican inhibit the activity of reverse transcriptase and induce a decrease of P24 antigen and an increase of CD4 cell number (Wu *et al.*, 1995). Three kinds of proteins, Alph-momordicine, Beta-momordicine and MAP-30, extracted from Momordica charantia, were found to be able to kill HIV-infected macrophage, and the number of CD4 cell was obviously increased (Zhang *et al.*, 1992). Extracts of Ganoderma Lucidum seu Japonicum were reported to have the effect of elevating expression of CD4 cell both *in vivo* and *in vitro* (Sunee *et al.*, 1992). Rhizoma Polygoni Cuspidati was found to have anti-HIV effect as well as inhibitory and killing effects on Staphylococcus Aureus, Streptococcus, Pseudomomas Aeruginosa, etc. (Jiang, 1995). The Japanese Fukuoka Institute of Environmental Health reported the results of their experimental studies on Spica Prunellae, Stigma Maydis and Radix Arnebiae. Stigma Maydis can prevent AIDS infection; spica Prunellae and Radix Arnebiae can inhibit the multiplication of HIV; and Phyllanthus urinaria L. has obvious anti-virus effect. It has a strong inhibitory effect on hepatitis virus, DNA polymerase and reverse transcriptase of AIDS virus (Zhou *et al.*, 1993). Japanese scholars confirmed the anti-HIV effects of Rhizoma, Radix Bupleuri, Rhizoma Smilacis Glabrae and Herba Hedyotis Diffusae, and discovered that Saikosaponin is a key factor in the effectiveness of Compound Radix Bupleuri Prescription (Wu, 1991b). Some scholars found that Salaspermic Acidin Radix Tripterygii Wilfordii and its derivatives have anti-HIV effects (Su *et al.*, 1992). Yang (1992) of the Taipei Hospital reported the anti-HIV effects of ingredients of Chinese drugs Folium Psidii Guajavae and another plant, the grape root. The Japanese Kobe Women Pharmacological University found that when extracts of fresh mushroom (1/100,000 g) was put into HIV-infected T cells, the virus was inhibited, and 97% of the cells were protected. The above-mentioned experimental studies indicate that a variety of Chinese medicine are able to inhibit the AIDS virus and can enhance the immunological function. Therefore, further extensive studies are warranted.

(2) *Studies on effective components of Chinese drugs*

Based on isolating, extracting and purifying Chinese drugs and studying their therapeutic action, many scholars found that each Chinese drug contains various kinds of compounds which play important roles in inhibiting the AIDS virus and enhancing the immunological function of the body. Experimental studies proved that polysaccharides, such as polysaccharides of Radix Ginseng, Glossogyne tenuifolia Cass, Radix Astragali, Ganoderma Lucidumsec Japonicum, Radix Actinidiae have enhancing immunity and regulatory effects. Algal polysaccharides can inhibit reverse transcriptase, sulphuric acid polysaccharide can inhibit HIV replication, and Glossogyne tenuifolia Cass polysaccharide is capable of competing target cell with HIV (Zhu, 1991; Li, 1994b; Zhang, 1944). Protein components have the double effect of regulating immunity and inhibiting HIV. For example, glucoprotein in Aloe can promote the increase of CD4 and macrophage, and induce the interferon and interleukin. A component from Radix Trichosanthis can kill the HIV-infected macrophage. Alpha and Beta Momordicines in Momordica charantia can cause inactivation of ribose. Ricin bond A has HIV inhibition effect (Liu *et al.*, 1994). Studies on Rhizoma cimigenol saponin revealed that it has SIV inhibition effect, reducing the production of SIV 2 to 3 units and the condition of cytopathy is alleviated (Liu *et al.*, 1994).

(3) *Studies on CM compound prescriptions*

Japanese scholars have discovered the inhibitory effect of Xiao Chai Hu Tang on reverse transcriptase and found the extract of Radix Acutellariae to have stronger effect and can inhibit PGE2 and the production of peroxide (Koji *et al.*, 1992). Masao *et al.* (1990) of the Tokyo Medical University discovered that Decoction of Ginseng could inhibit recombination of HIV, increase CD4 cell, exert inhibitory effect on CD8 cell, enhance activity of NK cell, and the metal element germanium in Radix Ginseng can raise the detoxifying function of the liver (Zhong *et al.*, 1990). The results of investigation on Kang Ai Zi Yi Hao (Anti-AIDS No. 1) proved the effectiveness of this remedy in raising activity of NK cell, raising the IL-2 level and the proliferative action of T cell (Zhu *et al.*, 1993). Furthermore, in some other experimental studies, Jin LiEr capsule, Hong Bao (An Ji Li Ke), etc. were all shown to have the effect of promoting the function of T cell, the activity of NK cell, and some even have HIV inhibition effect (Lu, 1997). Li (1990) screened

56 kinds of clinical commonly used injections of Chinese drugs by inhibition of HIV activity on H9 cell and MOLT-4 cell, and found that 10 kinds of drugs have an inhibitory effect on HIV infection. By comparing their 50% and 90% inhibitory dosage, it was found that the injection of Compound Radix Salvia Miltiorrhizae and the Yin Huang injection have the best effects.

11.3.2 *Experimental research of Chinese medicine on models of AIDS*

Studies on the influence of Chinese drugs on immunological function of the body and anti-virus action in animal models indicate that both single drugs and compound prescriptions have regulating immunity and anti-virus effect to a certain degree. Guan *et al.* (1993) in their experimental animal investigation, observed 112 cases of HIV/AIDS treated with clinical effective drug Glyke prescription and a total effective rate of 46.43% was obtained. The results of animal investigation indicate that the preparation has effects on mice with inhibited immunity, elevating the plaque formation test, specific rosette formation test, delayed hypersensitivity test and mixed lymphocyte cultivation test, increasing IL-1 and IL-2 levels and exerting inhibitory effect on SIV and HIV. Zhongyan No. 1 was used in the treatment of 110 cases of HIV/AIDS, and the total effective rate was 40%. In the models of SIV mac-infected monkeys with AIDS, the prescription was shown to have the effects of decreasing the titres of peripheral blood mononuclear cell and plasma virus, inhibiting AIDS virus and the activity of reverse transcriptase, increasing CD4 cell and CD4/CD8 value, and inducing the growth of interferon. Activation and proliferation of lymphocyte and renovation of damaged cells were identified in the pharmacological study. The results were superior to that of AZT control group (Guan *et al.*, 1995). The experimental study was also built up in SIV mac infected model monkey, the antiviral, immunomodulatory and pathological effect of ZY-I and ZY-II recipe was observed. The results showed that in comparing with AZT and control groups, the ZY-I could not only reduce the virus titer in plasma, inhibit the activation of HIV and reverse transcriptase *in vitro*, but also increase CD4 count and enhance the ratio of CD4/CD8.

The ZY-2 could reduce the viremia after 12 weeks of treatment and the P27 antigen of plasma was lowered from 122 pg/ml to 48 pg/ml, CD4 count was increased to near the normal level after 8 weeks of treatment. In addition, ZY-2 could also regulate the level of neopterin β_2-microgloblin in plasma. In the pathological examination, the author discovered that ZY-2 could activate and proliferate cells in lymph nodes. The above results suggested that prescriptions based on the principle of strengthening body resistance to eliminate pathogenic factors, could not only enhance the immune function mainly, but also inhibit the HIV to a certain extent. Experimental studies on animals provide evidence of clinical therapeutic effects of Chinese drugs in the treatment of AIDS (Guan *et al.*, 2003a).

11.4 Conclusion

AIDS is a viral infectious disease that endangers the health of mankind. After more than ten years of study, AZT, DDI, DDC, D4T, 3TC and protease inhibitor are found to be effective in the treatment of AIDS.

A combined therapy of several drugs (HARRT) was officially introduced to treat AIDS. The researches on AIDS have made great progress. But there are still problems of toxic effect, side effects and drug resistance. The more serious development is the rampant incidence of AIDS in Asia in recent years and the difficulty of most developing countries in meeting the cost of treatment. A lot of scholars have suggested to focus on the studies using alternative therapy. The study of TCM therapy has attracted worldwide attention. At present, studies of AIDS treatment with Chinese drugs require further development. It is especially important to design strict research schemes under the guidance of basic theory of TCM, control the prescription's standards of quality, adopt the international diagnostic standards and criteria for evaluating therapeutic results, conduct therapeutic evaluation of the effects of viral load volume and immunological function, and develop appropriate prescriptions for different stages and different conditions of the disease. We should spare no efforts to develop AIDS treatment using TCM and modern scientific approaches, and by combining Western and traditional Chinese medicine, so as to contribute to the prevention and treatment of AIDS and the welfare of mankind.

References

Alaka, K.D., *et al.* (1995) Clinical response of HIV/AIDS to alternative herbal medicine — a pilot study. In: *3rd International Conference on AIDS in Asia and the Pacific*, Thailand, October 1995 (Abstract PA 301).

Chang, R.S., *et al.* (1988) Screening anti-AIDS Chinese drugs. *Antiviral Res.* **9**, 163–176.

Chen, K.J. (1989) Clinical observation of treating AIDS with TCM. In: *Compilation of Theses of Synposium of AIDS and TCM*, July 1989.

Fu, L.N., *et al.* (1994) A report on 6-year follow-up observation of 3 cases of AIDS treated with TCM. *Zhejiang J. Tradit. Chin. Med.* **29**(9), 405–406.

Goh, M., *et al.* (1994) Herb tea treatment for AIDS patients in an AIDS nursing facility. In: *10th International Conference on AIDS*, Yokohama, August 1994 (Abstract PA 218).

Guan, C.F. (1993) Experimental study on screening anti-AIDS Chinese drugs with SIV. *Chin. J. Integr. Tradit. West. Med.* **13**(3), 162–164.

Guan, C.F., *et al.* (1993) Experimental investigation of treatment of AIDS with GLYKE. *J. Tradit. Chin. Med.* **34**(6), 365–367.

Guan, C.F., *et al.* (1995) Experimental investigation of effects of Zhongyan No. 1 on AIDS monkey models. *Chin. J. Infor. Chin. Med. Pharm.* **2**(5), 42–44.

Guan, C.F., *et al.* (2003a) Experimental study on treatment of SIV Mac-infection by Zhongyan No. 2. *Chin. J. Integr. Tradit. West. Med.* **9**(2), 156 (English edition).

Guan, C.F., *et al.* (2003b) Clinical and experimental study on treatment of HIV/AIDS patient by Zhongyan No. 2. *Chin. J. Integr. Tradit. West. Med.* **23**(7), 494–497.

Huang, B.S. (1990) *Treatment of AIDS with TCM*. Heilongjiang Scientific and Technological Publishing House, pp. 12–27.

Jiang, Y. (1995) A study on the effect of treatment of AIDS with Rhizoma Polygoni Cuspidati. *Dazhong Weisheng* **1**,14.

Jin, E.Y., *et al.* (1993) Antiviral effect of 12 kinds of Chinese traditional herbs against HIV-1 *in vitro*. *J. Ther. Res.* **14**(12), 251–253.

Khansari, N. and Mohraz, M. (1995) Effect of a medicinal plant extract on HIV and AIDS patients. In: *3rd International Conference on AIDS in Asia and the Pacific*, Chiang Mai, September 1995 (Abstract PA 305).

Koji, M., *et al.* (1992) Effects of Sho-Saiko-To (SST) PGE2, LTB4 and superoxide from peripheral monocytes and neutrophilis isolated from HIV infected individuals. In: *8th International Conference on AIDS*, Amsterdam, July 1992 (Abstract POA 2345).

Koji, M., *et al.* (1994) Potential role of traditional Chinese herbal medicine in treatment for HIV infection. In: *10th International Conference on AIDS*, Yokohama, August 1994 (Abstract PA 217).

Krishnamurthy, V., *et al.* (1995) Effect of Siddha medicine in the treatment of AIDS. In: *3rd International Conference on AIDS in Asia and the Pacific*, Thailand, October 1995 (Abstract PA 303).

Li, G.Q. (1994a) Experience in treatment of AIDS with principles of differentiation of syndromes. *Jiangsu J. Tradit. Chin. Med.* **15**(2), 53–55.

Li, M., *et al.* (1996) Study of Sheng Ming Quan to treat AIDS patients. *Chin. J. Prevent. Control STD AIDS* **2**(1), 26–28.

Li, S.Y. (1995) Preliminary clinical observation on treatment of AIDS with Qian Kun Ning. In: *'95 China International Symposium on AIDS*, Beijing, December 1995, p. 65.

Li, X.L., *et al.* (1990) *VI International Conference on AIDS* (ThA-237).

Li, Y.F. (1994b) Progress of anti-AIDS drugs. *Chin. Pharm. J.* **29**(12), 707–709.

Lin, X., *et al.* (1994) Inhibitory effect of Rhizoma Saponin on SIV *in vitro* and its mechanism. *West. Chin. Pharm. J.* **9**(4), 221–224.

Liu, Z.Y., *et al.* (1994) Research of natural products on anti-AIDS natural products. *Res. Dev. J.* **6**(4), 85–90.

Lu, W.B. (1997) Progress of treatment of AIDS with TCM. *J. Tradit. Chin. Med.* **38**(6), 368–371.

Lu, W.B., *et al.* (2002) Progress on treatment of AIDS by traditional Chinese medicine. *Chin. J. Integr. Tradit. West. Med.* **22**(10), 724–728.

Lu, W.B., Zhuang, J.D., Wu, B.P., *et al.* (1992) Treatment of 158 HIV-infected patients with traditional Chinese medicine in Dar Es Slaam, Tanzania. In: *Compilation of Theses for Practice of Treatment and Research on AIDS with TCM, Vol. 1.* People's Medical Publishing House, Beijing, pp. 1–6.

Luo, S.D., *et al.* (1996) Screening Chinese drugs with anti-AIDS effects. In: *11th International Conference on AIDS*, Vancouver, July 1996 (Abstract A25).

Masao, H. (1988) Therapeutic effect of minor decoction of bupleurum and decoction of ginseng for treatment of hemophilia patients with dysimmunity. *AIDS Ref. Mater.* **8**, 58–60.

Su, C.L. (1992) A report on 30 cases of AIDS treated by TCM. In: *Compilation of Theses for Practice of Treatment and Research on AIDS with TCM, Vol. 1.* Beijing People's Medical Publishing House, pp. 38–40.

Su, Y.K., *et al.* (1992) A study of the component of Radix Tripterygii wilfordii with anti-HIV effect Salaspermic Acidin and its derivatives. *Chin. Herb. Med.* **23**(7), 365.

Sunee, S., *et al.* (1992) Immunological regulatory effect of Ganoderma Lucidum seu Japonicum. In: *8th International Conference on AIDS*, Amsterdam, July 1992 (Abstract PB-3521).

Tan, X.S., *et al.* (1992) A study on screening anti-AIDS Chinese drugs with reverse transcriptase of AIDS virus and infectiousanemia virus. *J. Tradit. Chin. Med.* **3**, 39–41.

Wang, J., *et al.* (1994) Observation on 191 cases of HIV infection with ecchymosis on tongue proper. *J. Tradit. Chin. Med.* **35**(3), 156–158.

Wang, J., *et al.* (1995) Primary approach to treatment of AIDS with syndrome differentiation. *Acta Coll. Med. Guizhou.* **17**(4), 1–3.

Wu, B.P. (1991a) Experience of treating diarrhea of AIDS. *J. Tradit. Chin. Med.* **32**(12), 13–14.

Wu, B.P. (1991b) The study of prevention and treatment on AIDS with TCM. *Chin. J. Integr. Tradit. West. Med.* **11**(8), 497.

Wu, B.P., *et al.* (1995) Pharmacological study of Radix Scutellariae. *J. Tradit. Chin. Med.* **36**(6), 367–369.

Yamamoto, N. (1989) A study on pharmacological effects of Radix Glycyrrhizae. In: *International Informal Consult on AIDS*, Japan, February 1989.

Yang, L.L. (1992) Inhibitory effect of Folium Psidii guajavae on AIDS virus. *Infor. Chin. Med. Pharm.* **2**, 29.

Yoichi, G. (1988) Therapeutic effect of preparation of glycyrrhizin in treatment of AIDS. *Foreign Med. Sci. Tradit. Chin. Med. Sect.* **10**(4), 47.

Zhang, Q.C. (1990) Compound Q. *Ohai Press* **12**, 16–18.

Zhang, Q.C., *et al.* (1992) Purification and pharmacological effect of Momordica Charantia. *J. Naturop. Med.* **3**(1), 65–69.

Zhang, S. (1944) The study of the component of herbal medicine of anti-HIV activity. *Infor. Chin. Med. Pharm.* **4**, 30–33.

Zhao, S.Z. (1989) Experience of treating AIDS with TCM. *Zhejiang J. Tradit. Chin. Med.* **24**(10), 435–438.

Zhong, J.D., *et al.* (1990) *Treatment of AIDS with Chinese Medicine.* Shandong Science and Technology Publishing House, pp. 60–65.

Zhou, S.W., *et al.* (1993) Current situation of studies on pharmacological effects and clinical application of Phyllanthus Urinaria. *J. Chin. Pharm.* **28**(10), 589–592.

Zhu, B.F., *et al.* (1993) A study on a compound prescription of TCM Anti-AIDS No. 1. *Chin. J. Exp. Clin. Immunol.* **5**(4), 40–43.

Zhu, Y.L. (1991) Investigation of TCM and natural drugs on anti-AIDS. *J. Chin. Pharm.* **16**(12), 707–710.

Chapter 12

Research and Production of Dachengqi Granules

Xian-zhong Wu, Zai-shan Tian & Chang Chen

Abstract

Since the 1960s, Dachengqi decocation, being a representative recipe for purgative method, has been clinically used in surgical abdominal diseases with satisfactory results. Experimental studies have revealed the pharmacological effects of Danchengqi granules: increase of intestinal smooth muscle electric excitability; enforcing gut motility; increase of intestinal blood flow; protection of bowel barrier; inhibition of microbial and endotoxin translocation; inhibition of lesion Ca^{2+} inflow; reducing the size of endotoxin pool; inhibition of over production of cytokines; and inhibition of tissue peroxidation injury. Pharmaceutical research includes the composition, dosage, stability of raw material, selection of adjuvants and preparation form, identification, and toxicology study.

Keywords: Chinese Medicine; Acute Abdomen Purgative.

12.1 Introduction

As a representative recipe for purgative method of traditional Chinese medicine (TCM), Dachengqi Decoction is commonly used clinically in cleaning up the digestive tract, attacking the pathogenic factors, expelling stagnancy and clearing up heat toxins. Hence, it is indicated in fecal impaction in the gastrointestinal tract, interaction of pathogenic factors and heat, phlegm-dampness, blood stasis and other kinds of excess syndrome.

The purgation method can be traced to the ancient book *Canon of Medicine*, in which "Dispel or purgate inside the body if the epigastrium is full, and break the hard fecal matter first, and then expel the pieces" was recorded. In a later book, *Treatise on Febrile Diseases*, syndromes indicated or contraindicated for purgation were laid down; in addition, a series of modified prescriptions of Chengqi and Daxianxiong Decoction were suggested. The application of purgation became matured.

Since the early 1960s, the purgation method by herbal medicine has been used in China in the treatment of surgical abdominal diseases (Surgical Acute Abdomen Group, 1961). From the 1960s to the 1970s, it was mainly used in treating common acute abdominal diseases; experience in its usage was accumulated, forming a basis for further research. In the 1980s, the purgation method was also employed in the treatment of severe critical acute abdomen such as severe acute pancreatitis, and acute severe cholangitis. In the last decade, with the discovery of the phenomena of intestinal microbial and endotoxin translocation (Alexander *et al.*, 1990), the purgation method has also been used in the management of severe inflammatory reaction syndrome (SIRS)/multiple organ deficiency syndrome (MODS) with satisfactory results.

12.2 Background of Clinical Investigation and Experimental Research of Dachengqi Granules

The investigation and production of a new preparation should be built on the basis of definite clinical therapeutic result, which is the prerequisite and basis of prediction of the success of research and production. Our early work in this aspect has been firm and fruitful.

1. *As a main therapeutic principle in acute intestinal obstruction*

   Based on the theory of "the six viscerae are functioning when they are patent or unobstructed", and evidenced by multicentre, large-scale sample clinical observations, Dachengqi Decoction treatment in acute intestinal obstruction could have a success rate of around 70%, freeing from operation. In the recent two decades, 1199 out of 1484 cases (80.8%) of acute intestinal obstruction were cured by non-operative treatment, with a mortality of 2.7% (He *et al.*, 2001), while from 1961 to 1978, 2526 out of 3800 cases (66.5%) were successfully treated with a mortality of 3.5% (Tianjing Nankai Hospital, 1997).

2. *Purgation combined with other therapies used in abdominal inflammations*

   (a) Severe acute pancreatitis (SAP)

   The pathophysiology of SAP was not clearly understood until the 1980s. Hence, various therapies have been used. However, the mortalities of SAP all over the world were over 30%. Prospective studies were carried out — patients with SAP were analysed by syndrome differentiation of TCM and allocated into the initial, progression and recovery stages. In addition to systemic supportive management, the purgation method was used to reduce abdominal distention and maintain bowel movements by Dachengqi Decocation or Qingyi Xianxiong Decoction. In the initial stage (first 3 days after admission), more than 3 movements per day were expected. In the progression stage, control of infection and prevention of complication were emphasised, mainly by herbs that clear heat, detoxicate and activate blood circulation to dispel stasis effects, together with purgation. Appropriate remedies were then instituted in the recovery stage. In the series of 145 cases, nine patients died in the early stage and 15 in the progression stage. The overall mortality was 16.6% (24/143), which favourably compared to other reported studies (Cui *et al.*, 1999).

   (b) Acute severe cholangitis (ASC)

   Prior to the 1980s, the disease was treated mainly by emergency surgery, with a mortality of 10%–20%. Since the development of endoscopic nasal drainage (ENBD), the results were markedly improved (Hu *et al.*, 1989). From 1992 to 1995, a staging therapeutic regime was made up. After ENBD patients remained in distention and fever status for a period of time, Dachengqi granules were administered — two packs twice daily. Soon after the resumption of bowel movements, distention subsided with active peristaltic sounds, the patients were in the remission condition, and Huoxue Qingjie granules (herbs that activate blood circulation, clear heat and detoxicate) were the main treatment. Three to seven days later, in the recovery stage, the patients were treated by herbs that support vitality effect. During this period, 213 patients with ASC were admitted. Of them, 36 were operated with four post-operation deaths; 177 patients completed endoscopic sphincterotomy and ENBD treatment followed by herbal medicine; and two of them died. The overall mortality was 2.8% (6/213), which is lower than 4.8% (13/270) for the period of 1983 to 1990 (Hu *et al.*, 1989).

3. *Application of purgation in systemic inflammatory reaction syndrome (SIRS)/multiple organ deficiency syndrome (MODS) caused by severe abdominal infection*

   From 1993 to 1996, 295 patients with abdominal infection diagnosed as MODS were treated by integrated TCM and western medicine mainly through the therapeutic principle of purgation. Most of the patients were of APACHE-II 12 grades or over. Of them, 108 were conformed to multiple organ failure (MOF), APACHE-II more than 15 grades. On the basis of conventional effective therapy, the additional Dachengqi treatment led to prompt passage of flatus and stool, resulting in reduction of distention as well as improvement of peripheral circulation, of cardiopulmonary, liver and renal functions, and rapid decrease of plasma endotoxin, indicating the poly-level, multi-target visceral protective effects of purgation herbs (Cui *et al.*, 1996; Wu *et al.*, 2001).

4. *Pre-operative application of Danchengqi granules*

   Pre-operative administration of Danchengqi granules for the cleaning of G-I tract in patients with non-neoplasmic abdominal diseases might ameliorate post-operative inflammatory reactions, reduce the secretion of inflammatory media, and hence morbidities (Wang and Qi, 1999). The result of another study revealed that post-operative early administration of Danchengqi granules orally or by nasogastric tube if not contraindicated to those who underwent upper abdominal surgeries could move up the time of oral intake and of first post-operative bowel movement. Moreover, the lung functions (SaO2 and FEV1.0 (5PRED) were improved, plasma endotoxin level was lowered and motilin level elevated, indicating the prevention effect for enterogenic infection (Xie *et al.*, 2000).

5. *Experimental study of Dachengqi decoction*

   Experimental study revealed the following results: increase of intestinal smooth muscle electric excitability; enforcing gut motility; increase of intestinal blood flow; protection of bowel barrier; inhibition of bacterial and endotoxin translocation; inhibition of lesion Ca^{2+} inflow; reducing the size of endotoxin pool; inhibition of over-production of cytokines; and inhibition of tissue peroxidation injury. As a result, the lungs, kidneys, liver and other vital organs were protected from injuries by inflammatory factors (Wu and Tian, 1999; Zhi *et al.*, 2001).

12.3 Research and Production of Dachengqi Granules

The ancient recipe of Dachengqi decoction is composed of four components: rhubarb, magnolia bark, immature bitter orange and mirabilite. Since 1960, the decoction preparation has long been used in the treatment of acute abdominal diseases in this hospital. Continuous reform of preparation forms were made, in the form of concentrated decoction and of medicinal granules. The research and preparation of Dachengqi granules began in 1997 as an item of the National Science and Technology Major Study: Research on Standardisation of Compound Herbal Medicine — a joint initiative with Guangzhou University of Traditional Chinese Medicine.

Information on the chemical composition and on pharmacology and *in vivo* metabolism of the four composites of Dachengqi decoction were available. Based on conventional traditional Chinese medicine (TCM) theory, stressing the efficacy of the compound medicine as a whole, we tried to investigate the composition, quality, actions of the individual composites and the scientific connotation of the recipe, conformed the formal pharmaceutical norm on the basis of experimental and clinical studies, in order to produce safe, effective, good quality and controllable modern preparations of herbal medicine.

The prescription of Dachengqi granules is: Rhubarb 12 g; Magnolia bark 9 g; immature bitter orange 9 g; and sodium sulfate 4.5 g. Rheum palmatum L. (drug radix and rhizoma), Magnolia offincinalis Rehd, et Wils. var biloba Rehd. et Wils. (dark bark), Citrus aurantium L, cv. "choucheng" (immature fruit), and recrystallised dehydrated sodium sulphate were used as the raw material.

A pharmaceutical technological process was designed. It involves raw herbal material, extraction of individual herb, intermediate and product preparation, aimed at the homogeneity, quality controllability and ease of application of advanced production techniques.

Selection of adjuvants was based on the principle that the substance could lower the viscosity of Radix et Rhizoma Rhei to retain good purgative effect. Large amounts of mirabilite were used as another adjuvant. An antioxidant was added too.

Measurements were made on 11 components of Rhubarb anthroquinones, neosynephrine of Fructus Aurantii immaturus, magnolol and honokiol. Based on their content stability, the drying method for producing granules was determined.

Appropriate adjuvants were added into the intermediates (using extracts of Radix et Rhizoma Rhei and Magnolia bark, volatile oil of immature bitter orange and fine pure sodium sulphate) and then mixed. Under the designated temperature, granules of 20(m) were produced. The granules with specific smell and slightly sour taste were packed in aluminum-plastic packets (2.5 g/packet).

Identification was done by thin layer chromatography. Sodium ions and SO_4 ions were detected by chemical identification. HPLC showed magnolol and honokiol, sodium sulphate and other composites meeting the requirements stated in *China Pharmacopoeia 1995* edition, Appendix VI D.

12.4 Pharmacological and Toxicological Studies

Pharmacological studies revealed that Dachengqi granules markedly promote intestinal motion, effectively expelling endotoxin from the intestinal tract, reducing endotoxin translocation to plasma, decreasing plasma endotoxin contents, and exerting a favourable prevention and treatment effect of enterogenous endotoxemia following severe abdominal infection. Furthermore, Dachengqi granules significantly lower inflammatory media levels such as lipid peroxidase and NO, increase intestinal histaminase level, protecting the intestinal barrier. Acute toxicological tests in mice showed LD50 of Dachengqi granules as 24.63 g/kg, or 86 times of clinical dosage. Long-term toxicological tests in rats revealed no toxic effects after a 3-week administration of Dachengqi granules at a dose range of 1.72–6.90 g/kg (equivalent to six to 24 times of human dosage). Pathologic morphology revealed no adverse changes of the heart, lungs, liver, spleen, kidneys, brain, pituitary gland, thyroid, thymus and lymph nodes, adrenal glands, stomach, duodenum ilcum, pancreas, urinary bladder, testes, epididymis, prostate, ovary, uterus, bone and bone marrow of the animals, with a mortality of 0%.

Dachengqi granules are indicated mainly in enterogenous endotoxemia, or in TCM system: Yangming excess syndrome; heat bind with circumfluence; interior excess heat; dryness excess inner stool obturation and abiding food.

The dosage of the granules is as follows: two packets thrice daily for adults, and half the adults' dosage for children. They are to be administered orally with warm water.

In conclusion, the research and production of Dachengqi granules have been carried out consistently using TCM principles together with modern scientific techniques, an indication of moving toward herbal modernisation.

References

Alexander, J.W., Boyce, S.T., Babcock, G.F., *et al.* (1990) The process of microbial translocation. *Annu. Surg.* **212**, 496–512.

Cui, N.Q., Chi, Q.H., Kong, D., *et al.* (1999) Integrated medicine treatment in severe acute pancreatitis. *Chin. J. Surg. Integr. Med.* **5**(3), 129–132.

Cui, N.Q., Zhao, Q., Ge, Z.H., *et al.* (1996) Therapeutic results of purgation method in MODS caused by acute abdomen. *Chin. J. Surg. Integr. Med.* **2**(5), 315–320.

He, Q.Y., Zhou, Z.L., Wang, G.X., *et al.* (2001) Acute intestinal obstruction treated by integrated medicine, report of 1484 cases. In: *Symposium of VII National Conference on Clinical and Basic Studies of General Surgery 2001*, Tianjin, China, pp. 62–64.

Hu, J.S., Wu, X.Z., Lu, H.Z., *et al.* (1989) Clinical observation on ENBD and Qingjieling in treatment of acute severe cholangitis. *Chin. J. Integr. Med.* **9**(3), 144–147.

Surgical Acute Abdomen Group, Tianjin Medical College Affiliated Hospital, *et al.* (1961) Application of TCM purgation therapy in modern surgical treatment. *Chin. J. Surg.* **7**, 491–493.

Tianjin Nankai Hospital (1997) Acute intestinal obstruction treated by integrated medicine, report of 1006 cases. *Chin. J. Surg.* **3**, 139–141.

Wang, S.S. and Qi, Q.H. (1999) Effect of Dachengqi granules bowel pre-cleaning on serum inflammatory media of patients with acute abdominal diseases. *Chin. J. Surg. Integr. Med.* **5**(6), 385–387.

Wu, X.Z., Cui, N.Q., Zhao, Q., *et al.* (1981–2001) Application of purgation method in prevention and treatment of MODS. *Integr. Med. Tianjin* 2001, 117–119.

Wu, X.Z. and Tian, Z.S. (eds.) (1999) *Modern Research on Syndrome and Therapeutic Principles*. Tianjin Sci & Tech Translation Press, China, pp. 89–140.

Xie, J.L., He, Q.Y. and Xue, W.D. (2000) Clinical observation on post-operative early use of Dachenqi granules. *Chin. J. Surg. Integr. Med.* **6**(6), 384–386.

Zhi, L., Qiu, Q., Muladi, Cui, N.Q., *et al.* (2001) Therapeutic actions of Dachengqi granules on SIRS/MODS caused by enterogenous endotoxemia. In: *Symposium of VII National Conference on Clinical and Basic Studies of General Surgery 2001*, Tianjin, China, pp. 362–368.

Chapter 13

Study on Evacuation of Haematoma and Traditional Chinese Medical Therapy in Hypertensive Middle- and Large-Amount of Cerebral Haemorrhage

Mao-cai Liu, Pei-xin Huang, Yan Huang & Ming Lu

Abstract

This study examines the comprehensive therapeutic protocols of hypertensive middle- and large- amount of cerebral haemorrhage (HMLCH), and a scheme of study on combining evacuation of haematoma with traditional Chinese medical therapy. A series of clinical investigations were completed, e.g. investigation on the treatment of 201 cases with HMLCH by the comprehensive therapeutic protocols of traditional Chinese medicine (TCM) integrated with western medicine. The results showed that, compared with western medical management, the comprehensive therapeutic protocol showed more significant results in increasing survival rate and clinical curative effect, improving patients' quality of life and reducing complications. Some primary experimental mechanisms of the Chinese medicine were discovered: reduced the capillary permeability and brain water volume in model rats; cleared free radical; repressed the excessive production of NO while minimising its neurotoxic action; inhibited the excessive expression of cNOS mRNA and cNOS positive immunoreactive cells after cerebral haemorrhage; improved the expression of HSP 70 and HO-1; and protected neural tissue against injury.

Keywords: Cerebral haemorrhage; evacuation of haematoma; TCM therapeutics; laboratory study.

13.1 Introduction

The most common and important reason of cerebral haemorrhage is hypertension. Hypertensive cerebral haemorrhage, especially middle- and large-amount cerebral haemorrhage, is characterised by a high mortality and disablement rate — the reported mortality is 46%–99% among patients with routine medication and 67.1% among those with general operation (Yan *et al.*, 1996). With the aim of improving the clinical effect and to find a set of comprehensive therapeutic protocols for acute care, a therapeutic scheme was established on a basis of clinical facts and reviews of their therapeutic status quo. The concepts and methods of treatment, results of clinical investigations and some possible laboratorial mechanisms will be reported in this study.

13.2 Thoughts of Study

13.2.1 *Therapeutic status quo and analysis*

At present, the means for treating HMLCH include basic western medication, surgical therapy, Chinese herbal treatment and medical treatment based on traditional Chinese medicine integrated with western medicine.

The most heavily emphasised principles of internal medication and general management include: keeping the airway unobstructed, maintaining balanced nutrition, maintaining water-electrolyte and acid-base balance, preventing and treating cerebral oedema and/or cerebral hernia actively, preventing and managing complications zealously, regulating and stabilising blood pressure cautiously, promoting circulation, and expectant management, etc. (Chen, 1998; Shi, 1995; Wang, 2001). Doctors have focused on controlling temperature and blood sugar and decreasing blood pressure carefully (Lin *et al.*, 1999). As a strong osmotic diuretic, radical scavenger and cerebral preventive, mannitol helps resist cerebral oedema and reduce intracranial pressure. But a dehydrant is barely effective on patients with major haematoma and rapidly increasing intracranial pressure, and the quickly progressing cases. At the same time, doctors show great concern for its adverse effects (Feng *et al.*, 1997; Li, 1997). In cases of massive cerebral haemorrhage, a method of rapid effective medical treatment is still unavailable and mortality remains high (Han *et al.*, 1994; Qian and Zhang, 1996). Operation is an important way of first aid for patients with middle- and large-amount of cerebral haemorrhage. The wide application of CT and MR and the progression on microsurgery and stereotaxic techniques accelerated the development of operative treatment of cerebral haemorrhage and contributed to increase curative effect (Chen, 1998). Nevertheless, the mortality among severe cases remains high (Shi, 1995). Although an operation is able to clear haematoma and increase survival rates, the clinical effect is extremely influenced by dysfunction and digressive resistance secondary to acute space occupying effect and anaesthesia and operative injury, etc. (Hou *et al.*, 1989; Ma *et al.*, 1998). Also, post-operative complications present another set of problems.

Knowledge about cerebral haemorrhage was discovered quite early in the history of TCM. In the principle of diagnosis and treatment based on overall analysis of symptoms and signs, the therapeutic rules and prescriptions used to treat cerebral haemorrhage are variable. Among these, the rules of promoting blood circulation and removing blood stasis (活血化瘀), relaxing the bowels and removing heat (通腑泄热) are considerably effective. As traditional medical treatment may be ineffective for severe cases, the combination of TCM and western medicine is emphasised. The importance of TCM integrated with western medicine for treatment of cerebral haemorrhage is reinforced by recent clinical practice, especially in severe cases. The effect is more outstanding than not only TCM, but also western medicine and operation. So it is becoming an effective treatment method with great potential advantages for acute cerebral haemorrhage. Combining the principle of diagnosis and treatment based on an overall analysis of symptoms and signs in TCM with western medical treatment and expectant management may improve the effect. But the effect is still unsatisfactory in severe acute cases with massive haemorrhage. According to references on evacuation of haematoma and Chinese herbal treatment, TCM integrated with western medicine and the combination of internal medicine and surgical operation may manifest a more encouraging effect than internal treatment, but it is yet to be verified by further research (Liu *et al.*, 2001).

13.2.2 *Necessity and principles of comprehensive therapeutic protocols*

(1) In the treatment of HMLCH, the therapeutic methods of both TCM and western medicine have strengths and shortcomings. The same can be

said when comparing internal medicine and surgery. However, TCM integrated with western medicine has shown comparative advantages. Therefore, it is necessary to study comprehensive treatment using TCM integrated with western medicine. The pathogenic factors of hypertensive cerebral haemorrhage are multiple and complex. None of the existing therapeutic methods are able to eliminate all the factors. In order to get the best effect, comprehensive therapeutic protocols based on the organic combination of multiplex subjects should be present to match the complex pathogenesis of the disease with multiple taches, multiple levels and multiplex targets. Specialists like Silver have said that the combination of multiple subjects marked the modern treatment of stroke (Ming, 1997). Multi-subject comprehensive treatment is the fundamental and effective model for patients with HMLCH.

(2) Principles of Comprehensive Therapeutic Protocols

In order to use an organic combination of multiple therapeutic means to get the best effect, the following principles should be obeyed:

(a) Combine TCM with Western Medicine, and Learn from Others' Strong Points to Offset One's Weakness

Both TCM and western medicine have its own advantages and shortcomings. So we should use one's strengths to offset the other's weakness to gain more significant curative effect. It is useful to tap on the experience of western medical emergency measures for severe and urgent illness (e.g. to relieve space occupying effect by evacuation of haematoma and to reduce intracranial pressure) and microcosmic management (such as to maintain fluid-electrolyte and acid-base balance) for reference. On the other hand, the advantages of TCM such as diagnosis and treatment based on overall analysis of symptoms and signs, and holistic adjustment cannot be discounted.

(b) Retain the Characteristics of TCM, Develop the Holistic Adjustment of Prescriptions, and Increase the Effect

The foundation of Chinese herbal therapy is diagnosis and treatment based on overall analysis of symptoms and signs. So the method of treatment should be selected individually to match certain syndromes. In accordance with the syndrome, we can select the method of strengthening the body resistance, or eliminating pathogenic factor, or strengthening the body resistance and eliminating pathogenic factor at the same time. In that way, the clinical effect may be increased due to the development of the holistic adjustment of prescriptions.

(c) Grasp the Nature of the Disease, Combine Commonness with Specific Property

The reason and pathogenesis of HMLCH is complex. In clinical practice, we should grasp the nature of the disease. And the rules of treatment must be established to match the common reason and pathogenesis of the disease. Combine the specific property with the common property whenever it is possible.

(d) Be Simple and Clear, and Easy to Generalise

With the aim of making the cooperation and exchange between different departments and multiple subjects easier, the TCM syndromes and the therapeutic method should be simplified with characteristics of TCM. A simple and clear therapeutic protocol is easier to exchange and generalise.

13.3 Scheme of Study

13.3.1 *Selection of subjects*

The most common and important reason for cerebral haemorrhage is hypertension. More than 66%–77% of patients with cerebral haemorrhages are those with basal periganglionic haemorrhage. The special anatomic structure of basal ganglion and its importance in neural system determines the severity of the disease and the difficulty of emergency treatment and recovery. Bleeding of this site showed a higher mortality rate than others (Qian and Zhang, 1996; He and Guo, 1998). Clinical treatment for patients with middle- and large-amount of haemorrhage is difficult. We selected patients with hypertensive middle- and large-amount of basal periganglionic haemorrhage as subjects to establish and validate the therapeutic protocols. The study is not only representative, but also significant to clinical practice.

13.3.2 *Therapeutic protocol*

(1) Surgical Operation

The goals of surgical operation are clearing away haematoma promptly, decreasing intracranial pressure and relieving the symptoms, so as to buy time for the coming efficiency of comprehensive therapeutic protocol. Proper operations should be employed according to the situation of the patient, the condition of the hospital and the experience of the surgeon.

(2) Chinese Herbal Therapy

(a) Establishment of Therapeutic Principle

The therapeutic principles were established according to the main causes and pathogenesis of HMLCH as well as the main symptoms of excess syndrome and the possibility of clinical manifestations. Yang-excess syndrome, which characterises the domination of pathogen in acute period, is mostly caused by wind, fire, phlegm and blood stasis. Treating the incidence of an acute disease first is the principle. Clearing heat and calming the liver, removing blood stasis and phlegm, relaxing the bowels and restoring consciousness are the fundamental therapeutic methods for cases with Yang-excess syndrome. Yin-excess syndrome mostly manifests when the body resistance is weakened while pathogenic factors prevail. In such cases, eliminating pathogenic factors and strengthening body resistance is the principle. And the fundamental therapeutic methods include supplementing *qi* and promoting blood circulation, removing phlegm and obstruction in collaterals, relaxing the bowels and restoring consciousness.

(b) Selection of Chinese Herb

At present, no single drug solely represents the therapeutic methods for cases with excess syndrome in HMLCH. Corresponding to the complexity and variability of its pathogenesis, diversiform drugs with different routes of administration should be selected properly during comprehensive treatment.

Naomai II capsules, Tongfu Xinshen capsules and Qingkailing injection were selected for Yang-excess syndrome while Naomai I capsules, Tongfu Xinshen capsule and Ligustrazine injection for Yin-excess syndrome.

Naomai II capsules, Tongfu Xinshen capsules and Naomai I capsules are hospital preparations, the preparative technical flows proceeded in the light of uniform and orthogonal designs. Quality standards of the herbs included in the preparations were in accordance with the *Chinese Pharmacopoeia* (section 1, 1995 edition). Quality standards and chief items of identifications of finished products were established using identification and content measurement.

- Naomai II Capsules

  Ingredients: artificial Calculus Bovis; Cornu Babali; Radix Gentianae; Rhizoma Polygoni Cuspidati; Hirudo; Herba Leonuri, etc.

  Effects: remove heat from the liver and calm endopathic wind; remove blood stasis and phlegm; and induce resuscitation.

- Tongfu Xinshen Capsules

  Ingredients: Folium Cassiae; artificial Calculus Bovis; Rhizoma Polygoni Cuspidati; Semen Trichosanthis, etc.

  Effects: relax the bowels and remove heat; restore consciousness; and induce resuscitation.

- Naomai I Capsules

  Ingredients: Radix Astragali seu Hedysari; Rhizoma Ligustici Chuanxiong; prepared Rhizoma Arisaematis; prepared Rhizoma Gastrodiae; Herba Leonuri; prepared Rhizoma Pinelliae; Rhizoma Acori Graminei; Scorpio, etc.

  Effects: supplement *qi* and strengthen body resistance; remove blood stasis and phlegm; induce resuscitation; relieve convulsion; and spasm.

- Qingkailing Injection (produced by The Pharmaceutical Mill attached to Beijin University of TCM) to be developed on the basis of Angong Niuhuang Wan (Bezoar Bolus for Resurrection).

  Ingredients: Calculus Bovis; Cornu Babali; Pearl Powder; Radix Scutellariae; Flos Lonicerae; Radix Capejasmine; Radix Isatidis; Porcine cholalic acid; and Bovine cholalic acid (Cao, 1999; Research Group, 1975).

Effects: clear heat and purge fire; remove phlegm and the obstruction in collaterals; calm the liver to stop endopathic wind; tranquilise and allay excitement; restore consciousness and induce resuscitation; promote blood circulation and remove blood stasis, etc.

- Ligustrazine Hydrochloride Injection (produced by The Seventh Pharmaceutical Mill of Wuxi)

  Effects: promote blood circulation; and remove blood stasis in channels and collaterals.

  Indications: Yin-excess syndrome.

(c) Basic Treatment and Expectant Managements

This treatment includes: keeping the airway unobstructed; holding on balanceable nutrition; maintaining water-electrolyte and acid-base balance; preventing and treating cerebral oedema and/or cerebral hernia actively; preventing and managing complications zealously; regulating and stabilising blood pressure cautiously; expectant management; maintaining normal defection and urination; keeping the double-channel drainage tube or ventricular drainage tube unobstructed; proceeding with traumatic intracranial pressure monitoring if possible. Post-operative professional nursing include observing GCS, consciousness, pupil, drainage tube and vital signs.

13.4 Clinical Investigation

13.4.1 *Investigation on treating 201 cases with HMLCH by comprehensive therapeutic treatment of TCM integrated with western medicine*

(1) Clinical materials

(a) Source of Cases

All cases were the in-patients of The Second Hospital attached to Guangzhou University of TCM (Guangdong Provincial Hospital of TCM) and the cooperative units (Sino-Japan Friendship Hospital, The Third Hospital Attached to Guangxi Medical

University, Peoples' Hospital of Qinghai Province, The First Peoples' Hospital of Guangzhou City).

(b) Selection of Cases

Diagnostic standards: referred to the hypertensive diagnostic standard established by WHO in 1987 and The Diagnostic Outline of Cerebral Haemorrhage advanced in Chinese Medical Association, 2nd Countrywide Conference on Cerebrovascular Disease. All cases were diagnosed by CT or MR.

Diagnostic standard of stroke: referred to the diagnostic and therapeutic standard of stroke in therapeutic standards for medical emergency of TCM published by the National Administration Bureau of TCM in 1994.

All cases were accorded with the western medical diagnostic standards. And belong to stroke, apoplexy involving the solid organs with Yang-excess or Yin-excess syndromes separately. Age $\leq$ 80 years, course of disease $\leq$ 7 days, bleeding sited basal periganglion, amount of bleeding $\geq$ 30 ml, grades of consciousness situated II, III, IV according to *Cerebrovascular Diseases and Surgical Therapeutics* compiled by Wang Zhongcheng as editor-in-chief. Serious complications of heart, liver, kidney and so on were absent in all cases.

(c) General Conditions: a simple randomised control trial was applied in 201 cases, with 103 cases in the treatment group (T group) and 98 cases in the control group (C group).

The treatment group consists of 66 males and 37 females. Average age (years): 59.76 $\pm$ 11.97. Course of disease: 46 cases < 6 h; 31 cases 6–24 h; 26 cases > 24 h. Amount of bleeding: 53 cases 30–50 ml; 42 cases 51–80 ml; 8 cases > 80 ml. Mesal structural excursion: 71 cases < 5 mm; 22 cases 5–10 mm; 10 cases > 10 mm. Sixty-six cases with haematoma ruptured into ventricular and 13 cases with cerebral hernia. CT types of haemorrhage: 68 cases capsid; 35 cases external capsule and caudate nucleus. Consciousness: 47 cases lethargy; 38 cases shallow coma; 18 cases coma. GCS scores: 64 cases 3–9; 30

cases 10–12; 7 cases 13–15. Operations: 21 cases clearance of haematoma and depression by craniotomy with bone flap; 48 cases evacuation of haematoma with bone flap; 14 cases aspiration of haematoma integrated drainage with urokinase; 20 cases simple external ventricular drainage. The control group consists of 61 males and 37 females. Average age (years): 59.99 ± 8.56. Course of disease: 37 cases < 6 h; 38 cases 6~24 h; 23 cases > 24 h. Amount of bleeding: 42 cases 30~50 ml; 42 cases 51~80 ml; 14 cases > 80 ml. Mesal structural excursion: 68 cases < 5 mm; 25 cases 5~10 mm; 5 cases > 10 mm. Seventy-one cases with haematoma ruptured into ventricular and 18 cases with cerebral hernia. CT types of haemorrhage: 70 cases capsid; 28 cases external capsule and caudate nucleus. Conscious-ness: 42 cases lethargy; 42 cases shallow coma; 14 cases coma. GCS scores: 64 cases 3~9; 29 cases 10~12; 5 cases 13~15. Operations: 30 cases clearance of haematoma and depression by craniotomy with bone flap; 41 cases evacuation of haematoma with bone flap; 8 cases aspiration of haematoma integrated drainage with urokinase; 19 cases simple external ventricular drainage.

(d) Comparability Test Before Treatment

The insignificant difference between the two groups ($P > 0.05$) on gender, age, course of disease, amount of bleeding, GCS scores, consciousness, cerebral hernia occurring, mesal structural excursion, haematoma ruptured into ventricular, CT types, operative means and TCM syndromes as well as temperature, pulse, respiration, blood pressure, type of pulse, tongue condition and symptoms indicated the comparability between the groups before treatment.

(2) Therapeutic methods

(a) Treatment group: comprehensive therapeutic protocols

- Surgical operation
  Selected proper operation according to the situation of disease.
- Chinese herbal therapy guided with diagnosis and treatment based on overall analysis of symptoms and signs.

Apoplexy involving the solid organs with Yang-excess syndrome. Therapeutic methods: remove heat and calm the liver, eliminate blood stasis and phlegm, relax the bowels and restore consciousness. Drugs: (i) Tongfu Xinshen Xinshen capsules and Naomai II capsules. Took 4 capsules by nasal feeding after dissolving in warm boiled water and orally instead if the patient is awake, three times a day. The application of Tongfu Xinshen capsules lasted 10 d, reduced to half dosage for cases which defecated more than 5 times a day. And that of Naomai II capsules lasted 28 d. (ii) Qingkailing Injection 60 ml added into 500 ml of 5% glucose solution (for diabetic patients use normal saline instead), intravenous drip, once a day, lasted 28 d in all.

Apoplexy involving the solid organs with Yin-excess syndrome. Therapeutic methods: supplement *qi*, remove blood stasis and phlegm, remove obstruction in collaterals, relax the bowels and restore consciousness. Drugs: (i) Tongfu Xinshen capsules and Naomai I capsules. Took 4 capsules by nasal feeding after dissolving in warm boiled water and orally instead if the patient is awake, three times a day. The application of Tongfu Xinshen capsules lasted 10 d, reduce to half dosage for cases which defecated more than 5 times a day. And that of Naomai I capsules lasted 28 d. (ii) Ligustrazine hydrochloride injection 120 mg added into 500 ml of 5% glucose solution (for diabetic patients use normal saline instead), intravenous drip, once a day, 28 d in all.

- Basic Treatment and Expectant Managements

  This treatment includes: keeping the airway unobstructed, holding on balanceable nutrition, maintaining water-electrolyte and acid-base balance, regulating and stabilising blood pressure, preventing and treating complications such as pulmonary infection and haemorrhage of upper digestive tract etc., active and expectant managements etc.

(b) The control group

- Surgical operation

  Selected proper operation according to the situation of disease.

- Medical treatment
  Used mannitol according to the situation of disease: 20% mannitol 125–250 ml, intravenous drip, every 6 to 12 hours, reduced the dosage gradually. ATP 60 mg and coenzyme A added into 500 ml of 5% glucose solution (for diabetic patients use normal saline instead), intravenous drip, once a day, lasted 28 d.
- Basic treatment and expectant managements — similar to treatment group

(c) Standards of clinical effect assessment

After 28 d treatments, applied a 6-month follow-up survey on the patients. Referred to the standards of clinical effect assessment of cerebral apoplexy advanced in Chinese Medical Association, 2nd Countrywide Conference on Cerebrovascular Disease, the clinical effects was classified as nearly recovery (NR), obvious progress (OP), progress (P), without change (WC), depravation (DP) and death according to the improvement of neural function and the grade of disablement at the moment of assessment.

(d) Results

Refer to Tables 13.1 and 13.2 to see the clinical effects, and Tables 13.3 and 13.4 to see comparisons between groups on ADL.

Table 13.1. Comparison between groups on clinical effect after 28 d treatment.

Groups	n	NR (%)	OP (%)	P (%)	WC (%)	DP (%)	Death (%)
T group	103	4 (3.9)	24 (23.3)	52 (50.5)	12 (11.7)	0 (0)	11 (10.7)
C group	98	0 (0)	11 (11.2)	43 (43.9)	18 (18.4)	3 (3.1)	23 (23.5)

Rank test u = 3.922, P = 0.000.

Table 13.2. Comparison between groups on clinical effect after 6-month treatment.

Groups	n	NR (%)	OP (%)	P (%)	WC (%)	DP (%)	Death (%)
T group	95	19 (20.0)	35 (36.8)	28 (29.5)	0 (0.0)	0 (0.0)	13 (13.7)
C group	84	7 (8.30)	21 (25.0)	26 (31.0)	3 (3.6)	0 (0.0)	27 (32.1)

Rank test u = 3.639, P = 0.000.

Table 13.3. Comparison between groups on ADL after 28 d treatment.

Groups	n	0 (%)	I (%)	II (%)	III (%)	IV (%)	V (%)	VI (%)	VII (%)
T group	92	4 (4.3)	2 (2.2)	2 (2.2)	19 (20.7)	15 (16.3)	26 (28.3)	18 (19.6)	6 (6.5)
C group	75	0 (0.0)	2 (2.6)	1 (1.3)	7 (9.3)	7 (9.3)	24 (32.0)	25 (33.3)	9 (12.0)

Rank test u = 3.226, P = 0.002.

Table 13.4. Comparison between groups on ADL after 6-month treatment.

Groups	n	0 (%)	I (%)	II (%)	III (%)	IV (%)	V (%)	VI (%)	VII (%)
T group	82	19 (23.2)	7 (8.5)	11 (13.4)	18 (22.0)	7 (8.5)	15 (18.3)	4 (4.9)	1 (1.2)
C group	57	7 (12.3)	3 (5.3)	6 (10.5)	11 (19.3)	12 (21.1)	11 (19.3)	5 (8.8)	2 (3.5)

Rank test u = 2.242, P = 0.025.

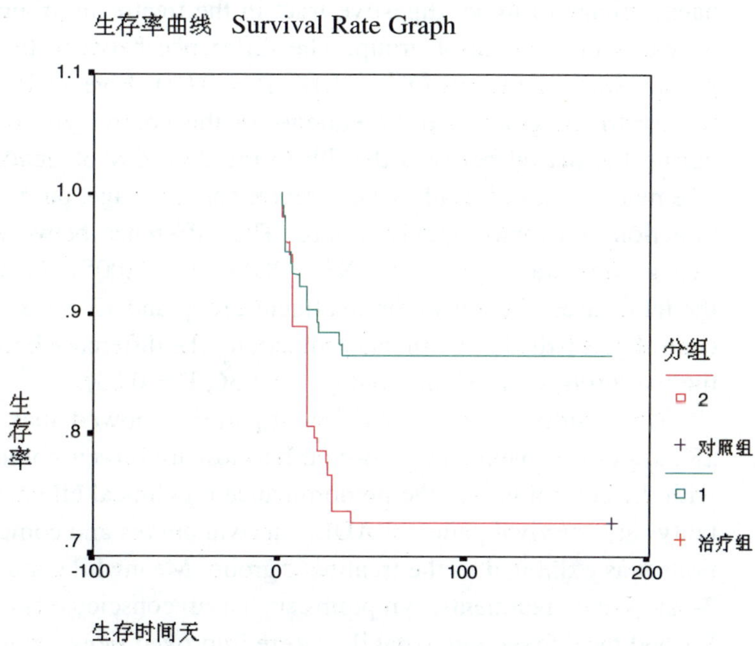

Figure 13.1. Comparison between groups on survival rate.

According to Fig. 13.1, the survival rate (green line) was higher in treatment group compared with the control group (red line), whereas the survival rate decreased rapidly in the control group. Data of the two groups were analysed by Kaplan-Merier survival estimates and Breslow test. The difference between the two groups was significant. Breslow = 6.46, $P = 0.011$.

After 3- and 7-day treatments, symptoms such as unconsciousness, rale, flushed face, fever and irritability were improved more significantly in the treatment group compared with the control group. The difference was significant ($P < 0.01$).

Fifty-four cases among the 103 patients in the treatment group manifested complications, compared to 75 cases among the 98 patients in the control group. Forty-five cases showed pulmonary infection in the treatment group and 66 cases in the control group. The difference between the two groups was significant ($X^2 = 11.37$, $P = 0.01$). Thirty-one cases showed haemorrhage of upper digestive tract in the treatment group and 43 cases in the control group. The difference between the two groups was significant ($X^2 = 4.10$, $P = 0.04$). Five patients in the treatment group and 17 patients in the control group died during the period between the 7th to the 28th day of treatment. The main causes of death were cerebral haemorrhage, pulmonary infection and multi-organic failure. The difference between the two groups was significant ($X^2 = 8.04$, $P = 0.005$). In all of the fatal cases, 5 cases in the treatment group and 13 cases in the control group died of pulmonary infection. The difference between the two groups was significant ($X^2 = 4.36$, $P = 0.03$).

The results of the above investigations showed that after 28 days of treatment and the 6-month follow-up survey, compared with the control group, the predominance on clinical effect, mortality rate, survival patients' ADL, survival curves and complications was exhibited in the treatment group. Meanwhile, after the 3- and 7-day treatments, symptoms such as unconsciousness, rale, flushed face, fever and irritability were improved more obviously in the treatment group compared with the control group, with a significant difference. All of these indicated the comprehensive therapeutic protocols, founded on the combination of evacuation of haematoma and Chinese herbal therapeutic in the guidance of diagnosis and treatment based on the overall analysis of symptoms and signs, benefits the patients much more than the simplex operative treatment and the western medical therapeutics.

13.4.2 *Effect of Naomai II capsules on cerebro-cardiac syndrome caused by cerebral haemorrhage*

Thirty-eight patients with cerebral haemorrhage, treated by Naomai II capsules, were brought into the investigation. All patients manifested abnormally in cardiac physicochemical examinations. The overall results and analysis showed that 30 cases among 38 patients with abnormal ECG were improved, and the general effective rate was 78.95%. Among the 18 patients with abnormal myocardial enzymogram, the amelioration of 14 cases indicated a general effective rate of 77.78%. This demonstrated the interferential actions of Naomai II capsules to the abnormal changes in ECG and myocardial enzymogram secondary to cerebral haemorrhage. Whether or not the patients had hypertensive history, unconsciousness and basal periganglic haemorrhage, the curative effect would not be influenced distinctly. But the effect was more outstanding in the patients without cardiopathic history and those with amount of bleeding less than 30 ml. And this suggested the possibility of a comparatively severe secondary cardiac injury may exist in patients with cardiopathic history and massive cerebral haemorrhage. Naomai II capsules helps to regulate the abnormal changes in ECG and myocardial enzymogram in the patients with cerebro-cardiac syndrome caused by cerebral haemorrhage.

13.4.3 *Influence of rectal drip with Tongfu Xinshen liquid on situations of consciousness in patients with coma secondary to haemorrhagic stroke*

In the basis of realisation of the effect of Tongfu Xinshen capsule in patients with cerebral haemorrhagic coma, a randomised control trial was applied in 61 patients in accordance to trial standards. The cases were divided into treatment group (n = 31) and control group (n = 30). Along with the general treatment, the patients in treatment group were given Tongfu Xinshen capsules by rectal drip, and the patients in the control group were given by nasal feeding. The treatment lasted 7 days. The pre-treatment comparison between the two groups on general conditions suggested the equivalence of their baseline. A comparison on time needed to restore consciousness between the two groups revealed that less time was needed in the treatment group. The difference between the groups was significant ($P < 0.05$). The scores of coma increased faster in the treatment group than in the others. The difference between the two groups was significant ($P < 0.01$). Scoring the neurofunctional damnification of the patients after 14 days of treatment, although the outcomes showed a higher effective rate of 80.65% in treatment group and a lower effective rate of 54.84% in the control group, the difference between them was insignificant ($P > 0.05$). Rectal drip with Tongfu Xinshen liquid, displayed the ability to accelerate the recovery of consciousness and minimise coma. This seemed like an effective way of treating coma in the acute stage of cerebral haemorrhage, and is worthy of further studies.

13.5 Laboratory Study

13.5.1 *Study of Tongfu Xinshen capsules, Naomai II capsules and Naomai I capsules on the possible precautionary and therapeutic mechanism in rat with cerebral haemorrhage*

Rat models with renal vascular hypertensive cerebral haemorrhage were established by occlusion of bilateral renal arteries and injection of collagenase, and then were treated respectively with Tongfu Xinshen capsules or Naomai II capsules or Naomai I capsules. The result showed that all the three preparations displayed effects in reducing the permeability of cerebral capillaries and brain water volume in different degrees, but Tongfu Xinshen capsules showed the most significant effect. Naomai II capsule and Tongfu Xinshen capsules improved the neural symptoms in rat models. Meanwhile, more uniform actions of the three preparations were observed in rat models, such as improvement of micro-circulation and the absorption of haematoma, protecting neuron against injury and promoting the restoration of neural tissues and the recovery of neural functions. In addition to the above-mentioned experiments, some in-depth laboratory studies should be present to match the complex pathogenesis of the vith multiple taches, multiple levels and multiplex targets. The ts can be achieved by combining traditional Chinese medicine tern medicine, while learning from each type's advantages to the other's shortcomings. The study approached the comprehenerapeutic protocols in 201 cases, and the results indicated the improved the clinical effect and reduced mortality for patients le- and large-amount of hypertensive cerebral haemorrhage, and the quality of life at the same time.

ent kinds of complications occurred in the majority of the postpatients with HMLCH. The number and the degree of the comare extremely important to the prognosis. Complications are reasons for the post-operative deaths in patients with cerebral age and the influencing factor to the recovery of the neural injury. The comprehensive therapeutic protocols decreased the rate of complications and the fatality rates in patients with cerebral haemorrhage and pulmonary infection. These may be ion with the holistic adjustment of the Chinese medicine adjust e of viscera, Yin and Yang, as well as blood and *qi* by diagnosis ent based on overall analysis of the symptoms and signs. Holistic t is the spirit of traditional Chinese medicine and is of great effects. Studying the rules of syndromes and therpeutics of post-operative patients is very important in looking for the sive therapeutic protocols and improving the effects.

e importance of two therapeutic methods in chief: xing the bowels and restoring consciousness, ting blood stasis and phlegm at the same time

ng the bowels and restoring consciousness

e patients with middle- and large-amount of cerebral haesuffered from constipation or dyschesia in the acute stage, or the serious cases. Combining with turbid pathogenic factors, fire accumulated in yangming, then turbid *qi* climbed up brain from the collaterals stomach to disturb the mental

were carried out to discover the mechanisms
The results substantiated that all the three
content of SOD in model rats' cerebral tissues
repress the excessive production of NO to mi
inhibit the excessive expression of cNOS
immuno-reactive cells to after cerebral haer
the influence of two different routes of admi
capsules on the expression of heat-stroke pro
haemorrhagic cerebral tissues was observec
stration improved the expression of HSP
effects in protecting neural tissues from inj
with rectal drip was better than the others.

13.5.2 *Study of Zhongfeng Jiedu decoctic precautionary and therapeutic mec cerebro-visceral syndrome seconda*

Rat models with cerebral haemorrhage we
collagenase, and then brought into the prin
ment of Zhongfeng Jiedu decoction (Rhizor
Calculus Bovis, Cornu Babali, Radix Notog
Rehmanniae, Radix Astragali seu Hedysari
as plasma concentration of lactic acid,
volume and pulmonary oedema were decre
acid was depressed ($P < 0.05, 0.01$). Th
and therapeutic mechanisms of it in rat
secondary to cerebral haemorrhage.

13.6 Discussion

13.6.1 *Comprehensive treatment based of multiplex subjects is the key t*

The pathogenic factors for severe patient
of cerebral haemorrhage are multiple and
sive therapeutic protocols based on the c

subjects
disease
best effe
with we
overcom
hensive
protocol
with mic
increase
Diffe
operative
plication
importan
haemorrh
functiona
incidence
recurrent
in connec
the balan
and treatr
adjustme
benefit tc
TCM in
comprehe

13.6.2 *Th re tre*

(1) Relax
Most of
morrhage
especially
pathogeni
toward th

activity. With excessiveness of earth and exhaustion of water, the fire-heat damnified Yin then aggravated the deficiency of Yin, excessiveness of fire and occurrence of wind. At the moment, the goals of removing fire-heat, sending down turbid, saving the kidney Yin, and restoring consciousness cannot be achieved without relaxing the bowels. We select Tongfu Xinshen capsules in clinic, to relax the bowels and relieve constipation with Folium Cassiae, Rhizoma Polygoni Cuspidati and Semen Trichosanthis, to remove heat, relieve toxin, restore consciousness and induce resuscitation with Artificial Calculus Bovis. The results of our laboratory study indicated Tongfu Xinshen capsules reduced the permeability of cerebral capillaries and brain water volume and improved the neural symptoms significantly.

(2) Treating blood stasis and phlegm at the same time

Blood stasis and phlegm, created through the course of stroke, are key pathogens of the disease. So we brought forward the rules of treating blood stasis and phlegm at the same time. In TCM, the blood that got out of the vessels is blood stasis. We emphasise the removal of blood stasis and phlegm as early as in the acute stage. When blood stasis and phlegm are removed, they cannot combine with fire-heat and the liver-wind, and this helps to send down fire and calm wind. For example, we select Hirudo and Herba Leonuri to remove blood stasis and promote blood circulation, and Sargassum to remove phlegm and induce resuscitation. It can be observed that both Herba Leonuri and Sargassum have natriuesis, and have certain effect on reducing cerebral oedema. According to our clinical experience, the removal of blood stasis and phlegm can accelerate the recovery of consciousness and the absorption of the haematoma, and improve symptoms such as rale, retraction of the tongue, and acroparalysis, etc.

(3) Analysis of TCM syndromes in HMLCH

Among 201 patients with excess syndrome of HMLCH, there are 184 cases of Yang-excess (91.54%). The percentage was congruent with figures reported (80%–95%) in references (collected 19 pieces, including 1201 cases with excess syndrome, among these, 1043 cases with Yang-excess syndrome, 158 cases with Yin excess syndrome). This indicated that the sample was representative. We summed up the references and the primary results of our investigations, and then considered that Yang-excess syndrome was the main type of syndromes of HMLCH in the patients with excess syndrome. But Yin-excess syndrome was not common in clinic: among 201 cases, there were only 17 cases. It probably involved the pathogenic characters (such as wind, fire, phlegm and blood stasis) of excess syndromes in HMLCH. Meanwhile, some patients died before arriving at the hospital, and some changed into collapse syndrome. All these may be important reasons that explain why Yin-excess syndrome is uncommon, while Yang-excess syndrome is most common in clinics.

In our study on TCM syndromes, we collected data on Yang-excess and Yin-excess syndromes simultaneously. Although Yin-excess syndrome was uncommon, some of them changed into collapse syndrome and the prognosis was relatively bad. We stress the establishment and the practice of comprehensive therapeutic protocols, while paying less attention to the study of standards of syndrome. Because Yin-excess syndrome is lacking, further investigations are needed for the treatment of such a syndrome.

References

Cao, X.L. (1999) The research of Qingkailing injection on stroke. *J. Emerg. Syndr. Chin. Med.* **9**, 176–181.

Chen, H.Z. (1998) *Practice Internal Medicine.* People's Medical Publishing House, Beijing.

Feng, X.P., Lu, Y. and Gong, X.L. (1997) The adverse reaction of mannitol in 695 cases with hypertensive cerebral haemorrhage. *Chin. J. Pharm.* **17**, 525.

Han, Q., Qi, L.P. and Zhang, Y.X. (1994) The cause of death of hypertensive cerebral haemorrhage treated conservatively and surgically: a comparative analysis in 357 cases. *Chin. Crit. Care Med.* **6**, 217–219.

He, Y.Q. and Guo, X.Y. (1998) The treatment device of serious putaman bleeding on CT. *J. Ningxia Med.* **20**, 99–100.

Hou, J.S., Lian, Z.G., Han, Q.S., *et al.* (1989) Clinical analysis of 157 cases postoperative complication of hypertensive cerebral haemorrhage. *Chin. Nerv. Ment. Dis.* **15**, 349–353.

Li, L. (1997) Measurement analysis in documents of mannitol on 620 cases. *Chin. J. Pharm.* **6**, 153–155.

Lin, C.S., Wang, H.X., Zhu, C.H., *et al.* (1999) The new progress of internal medicine on hypertensive cerebral haemorrhage. *J. Clin. Med.* **19**, 43–45.

Ma, Y.H., Zhan, R.Y., Zhou, Y.Q., *et al.* (1998) The analysis of prognostic factors in hypertensive basal ganglion haemorrhage with early surgery. *J. Zhejiang Med.* **20**, 454–456.

Ming, Z. (1997) Cooperation in multiple medical science is the notation of therapy on modern stroke. *Chin. Med. Trib.* **23**, 1.

Qian, H.S. and Zhang, G.Q. (1996) The new progress of fundamental and surgical treatment on hypertensive cerebral haemorrhage. *Cerebrovasc. Dis. Foreign Med. Sci.* **4**, 155–157.

Shi, Y.Q. (1995) *Practice Neurology.* Science and Technique Publishing House, Shanghai.

The Research Group on Peaceful Palace Bovine Bezoar Pill in Department of Chinese Medicine in Beijing College of TCM (1975) The research on new preparation on Peaceful Palace Bovine Bezoar Pill. *J. New Chin. Med. Pharm.* **8**, 12–13.

Wang, W.Z. (2001) *Neurology Cerebrovascural Diseases.* People's Medical Publishing House, Beijing.

Yan, H.F., Gong, Y.Y., Zuo, H., *et al.* (1996) Curative effect of hypertensive cerebral haemorrhage treated conservatively and surgically: a comparative analysis. *J. Brain Nerv. Dis.* **4**, 152.

Liu, M.C., Huang, P.X. and Liang, W.X. (2001) Thoughts of establishing comprehensive therapeutic protocols for hypertensive middle- and large-amount cerebral haemorrhage. *J. Guangzhou Univ. Tradit. Chin. Med.* **18**, 1–7.

Chapter 14

The Conceptual Framework of the Chinese Quality of Life (ChQOL) Instrument

Li Zhao, Kelvin Chan, Kwok-fai Leung, Feng-bin Liu & Ji-qian Fang

Abstract

When a new health-related quality of life (HRQOL) instrument is designed, it is important to develop the conceptual structure of the model during the process of development. The newly developed Chinese quality of life instrument (ChQOL) — a new generic HRQOL instrument — should be more sensitive in detecting the efficacy of Chinese medicine and supplementing the existing generic HRQOL instruments. This paper discusses the conceptual modeling in setting up the ChQOL based on the health concepts and practice of Chinese medicine.

Keywords: Chinese Quality of Life Instrument (ChQOL); Chinese Medicine; Health-Related Quality of Life.

14.1 Introduction

Quality of life (QOL) is generally considered to be one of the most important patient outcome measures in clinical trials, assessing effectiveness of treatment and research on quality of care. Increasingly, new evidence supports the importance of including patients' assessment of their health-related quality of life (HRQOL) in clinical studies. This trend makes it all the more necessary to have a clear methodology for the development and use of HRQOL instruments.

Chinese Medicine (CM) has been practised for thousands of years in China based on experience passed down from generation to generation. In the 1950s, because of national need, CM was officially re-introduced and integrated with orthodox (western) medicine as the mainstream medical care (Chan, 2002). Nowadays, not only has CM been utilised in primary health care in China, but it has also been applied in some developed countries as one of the complementary or alternative medicine where orthodox medicine is predominant in their national health care systems (Chan and Lee, 2002). With the tremendous expansion in the use of CM worldwide, the safety, efficacy as well as quality control of Chinese herbal medicines and traditional procedure-based therapies such as acupuncture have become key concerns for both health authorities and the public (Chan and Lee, 2002).

The challenge now is to ensure that CM is used properly and to determine how clinical research and evaluation of CM should be carried out. The recently emerged QOL research, as a new and relatively general approach for assessment, can possibly be used to evaluate the efficacy of clinical treatment in traditional medicine (World Health Organization, 2000). But QOL assessment for traditional medicine has received much less attention in the literature. This is because of difficulties in assessing the concepts of traditional medical practices such as CM according to the standards in the practice of western medicine. It is also problematic to determine which aspects of QOL CM should be involved. Translating the various domains and components of QOL into a quantitative scale is a complex task. Most QOL instruments consist of questionnares, some of which measure only a simple aspect of QOL. Other aspects such as psychological dimensions are complex and require more sophisticated measurements (Fayers and Machin, 2000; Fayers and Hand, 1997).

Many experts in Chinese medicine and psychometric scale development had expressed their views on the need of developing separate QOL instruments specific to Chinese Medicine. It was suggested that there is an urgent need to develop such HRQOL instruments based on the premises that the concepts of health in Chinese medicine are different from those developed according to the western medical practice (Liu *et al.*, 1997; Zhang and Wang, 2000). Hence, it is feasible to develop a new generic HRQOL instrument that is more sensitive and appropriate for the assessment of the efficacy of Chinese medicine (Zhang and Wang, 2000; Zhao and Chan, 2003), such as the Chinese quality of life (ChQOL) instrument that we began to develop.

In general, before embarking on developing a questionnaire for QOL assessment, the research questions should be formulated clearly. This will include the assessment of working definitions of what is meant by QOL, health concepts of CM and hypothetical models. It is envisaged that hypothetical models developed should maintain theoretical consistency, and, the postulated model should subsequently be adjusted to improve its fitness statistically (Bollen and Scott, 1993; Byrne, 1998; Kelloway, 1998; Scientific Advisory Committee of the Medical Outcomes Trust, 2002).

14.2 Conceptualisation of the ChQOL

Due to the lack of a universally agreed definition of QOL, the first step in the development of the ChQOL is to define the concept of QOL. In this paper, we have accepted the concept of QOL as defined by the World Health Organization (WHO), which interpreted QOL as an individual's perceptions of their position in life in the context of the culture and value systems in which they live and in relation to their goals, expectations, standards and concerns (World Health Organization, 1993). The QOL is a subjective appraisal of an individual of his/her life as a whole or various domains of his/her life. Such a subjective nature of QOL is widely adopted in the medical field.

14.2.1 *Health concepts of CM*

Presently, there is no QOL concept in CM. But the root of health concepts in CM, the theory of Yin and Yang (the core philosophy of Chinese medicine), can embody the QOL concept. A perfect *Equilibrium State* of Yin and Yang (阴阳平衡) reflects a perfect health state and implies a perfect state of life quality.

The *Equilibrium State* of Yin and Yang can be manifested in three dimensions. These are: the *harmonisation of physical form and vitality* (形神统一); the *harmonisation of man and nature* (人与自然统一), and the *harmonisation of man and society* (人与社会统一). The concept of

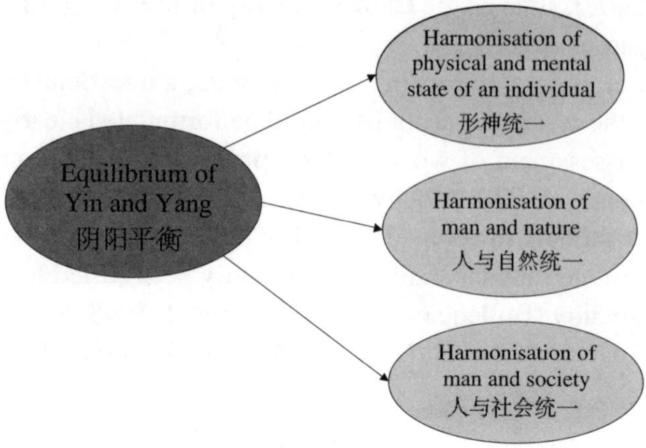

Figure 14.1. The basic requirements of ChQOL when applying the concepts of Chinese Medicine.

the *Equilibrium State* of Yin and Yang embraces the health concept suggested by the WHO completely. Health is a state of complete physical, mental and social well-being, and not merely the absence of disease or infirmity (World Health Organization, 1958). This is the basic framework of the ChQOL (Fig. 14.1).

The *harmonisation of physical and mental state* is one of the basic theories of CM. Physical form is the physical appearance, human body, physique or constitution including body build, complexion, stamina, etc. Vitality is the generalisation of all the physiological activities of the human body. It can reflect normal or abnormal life activities. But vitality cannot be severed from the physique alone. There can be vitality only when the physique exists. Sound vitality comes from strong physique and weak physique results in declined vitality. Vitality can be distinguished in a broad or narrow sense. Vitality in a broad sense refers to the total external manifestations of life activities of the human body that is the reflection of visceral functions. Vitality in a narrow sense refers to the mental activities including consciousness and thought processes of the human being (Fig. 14.2).

Both the harmonisation of physical form and vitality, and the harmonisation of man and nature are relevant to the quality of life. The

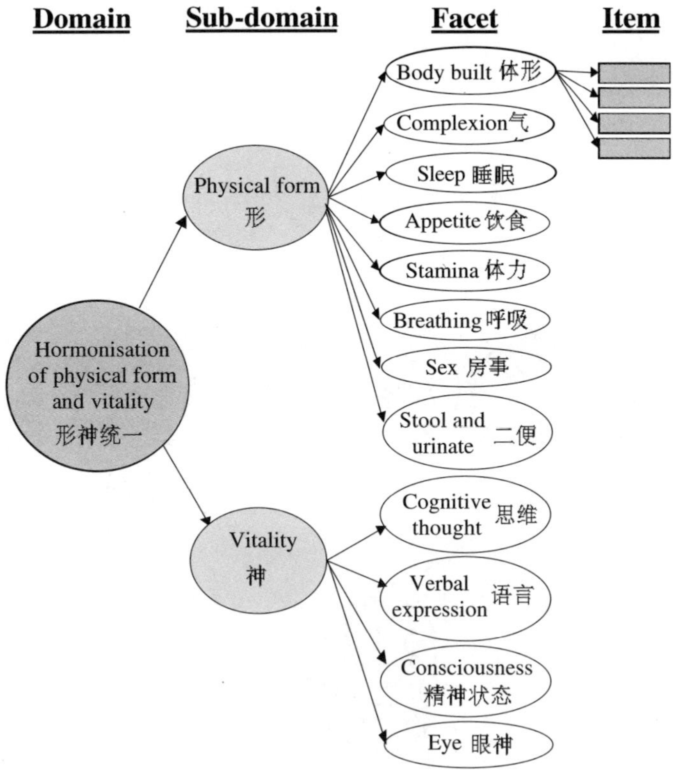

Figure 14.2. Harmonisation of physical form and vitality.

natural environment and conditions are the material basis for human survival. The movement and changes of nature have a direct and indirect influence on humans, who keep in touch with the natural environment through various sensory organs and adjust physically or psychologically to maintain homeostasis of the functioning body. These natural factors include season, climate and geographical environments.

Finally, man and society also demonstrate the harmonised relationship, because man is a part of society. Man should retain the adaptation and unity between himself and society by means of self-regulation and self-control. The social factors include family, work and personal relationships.

On the other hand, the *Theory of Seven Emotions* should be included as one of the basic theories of CM. The *Seven Emotions* refer to human

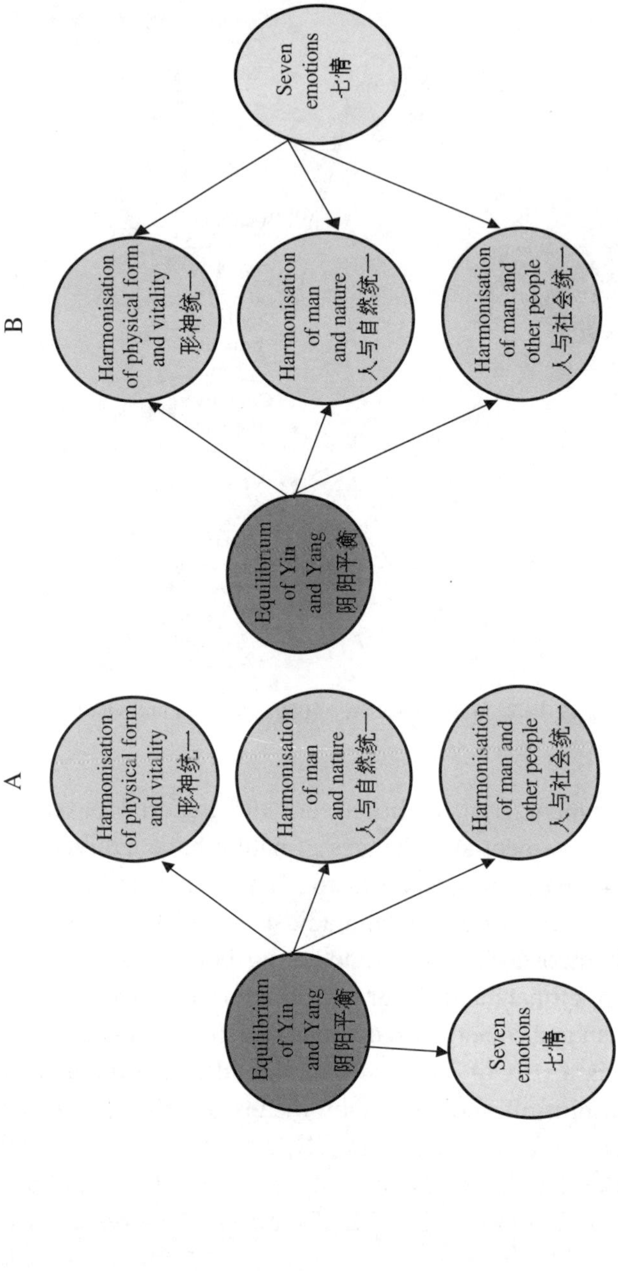

Figure 14.3. Structural relationship of *Seven Emotions* and *Equilibrium of Yin and Yang*.

emotions, which include anger, joy, worry, pensiveness, grief, fear and fright. The emotions can be regarded as psychological consequences of the interactions of the individual with the external environment including human and natural surroundings, and also as indicators of the internal health conditions of the individual. Under general circumstances, *Seven Emotions* are considered as normal psychological activities. However, when the *Seven Emotions* are beyond the normal range, the individual may experience imbalance or impairment of Yin and Yang, as well as *qi* and *blood*. This may lead to further pathological conditions. Therefore we have to accept the *Theory of the Seven Emotions* as one of the basis for the development of the ChQOL. Two possible relationships between the *Theory of the Seven Emotions* and the *Equilibrium of Yin and Yang* are illustrated in Fig. 14.3.

14.2.2 *The hypothetical model of ChQOL*

Figure 14.4 shows the proposed final structure of the ChQOL. Such a structure has similar features to many QOL instruments in the west. The "harmonisation of physical form and vitality" is an analogy with the physical or functional domain, the "harmonisation of man and nature" is an analogy with the environmental domain, and the "harmonisation of man and society" is an analogy with the social domain. The *Seven Emotions* can be used as an analogy with the psychological domain.

In developing a measuring instrument (questionnaire), a structure reflecting the concepts to be measured has to be constructed. It is desirable to include the theories in CM in the domain and facet structure so that the psychometric rules and statistical methods can be applied in the development of the ChQOL. These models serve as the starting point of our study. They will be further debated and scrutinised among theorists of CM before final model(s) can be established. Questions will then be drafted for each model and be used in field tests. The validity and relative advantages of the models and the psychometric properties of the questions will be tested empirically during the field studies.

This paper highlights the need for developing a conceptual structural model for the ChQOL. The remaining technical issues are related to the

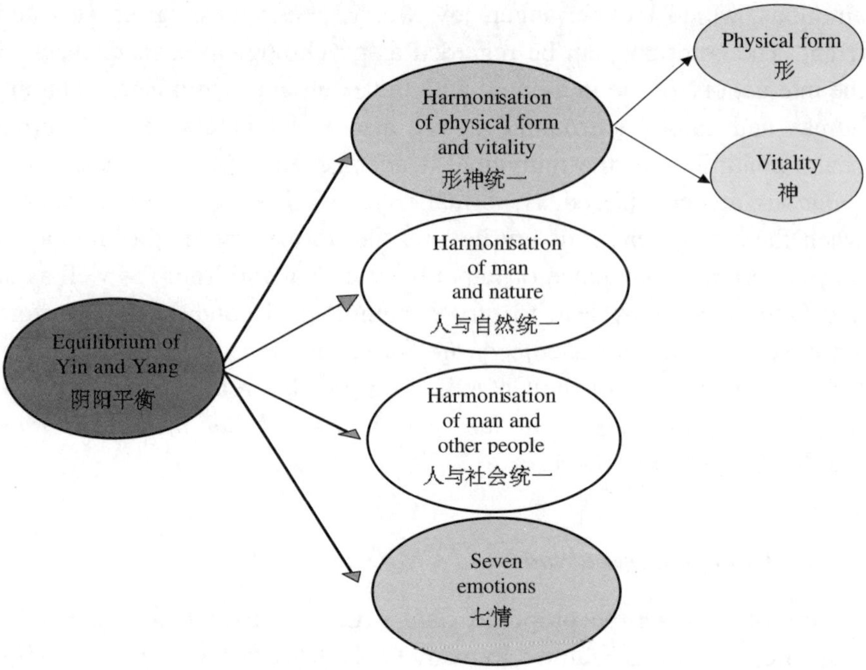

Figure 14.4. The final structure of the ChQOL model.

methodology of developing a high quality health status instrument, which can be accepted and adopted worldwide for Chinese medicine research. This is especially important when we want to incorporate the holistic balanced view of health in Chinese medicine into the instrument. It will also provide the foundation for future hypothetical models concerning the relationships between the items used in the instrument and the postulated domains of QOL, which can be then explored, tested and constructed for validity.

Acknowledgements

The project was partially supported by Faculty Research Grant of Hong Kong Baptist University (FRG/02-03/I-32).

References

Bollen, K.A. and Scott, L.J. (eds.) (1993) *Testing Structural Equation Models.* Sage Publications, Newbury Park, CA.

Byrne, B. (1998) *Structural Equation Modeling with Lisrel, Prelis, and Simplis.* Lawrence Erlbaum Associates, Mahwah, New Jersey.

Chan, K. (2002) The historical evolution of Chinese medicine and orthodox medicine in China. In: *The Way Forward for Chinese Medicine*, (eds.) Chan, K. and Lee, H. Taylor and Francis, London and New York, pp. 1–21.

Chan, K. and Lee, H. (eds.) (2002) *The Way Forward for Chinese Medicine*, (eds.) Taylor and Francis, London and New York.

Fayers, P. and Hand, D.J. (1997) Factor analysis, causal indicators and quality of life. *Qual. Life Res.* **6**, 139–150.

Fayers, P. and Machin, D. (2000) *Quality of Life — Assessment, Analysis and Interpretation.* John Wiley & Sons, West Sussex, England, pp. 1–3.

Kelloway, E.K. (1998) *Using Lisrel for Structural Equation Modeling — A Researcher's Guide.* Sage Publications, Thousand Oak, CA.

Liu, F.B., Wang, J.H. and Chen, W.W. (1997) The application of quality of life in Chinese medicine research. *New Chin. Med. Clin. Pharmacol.* **8**(3), 179–181.

Scientific Advisory Committee of the Medical Outcomes Trust (2002) Assessing health status and quality of life instruments: attributes and review. *Qual. Life Res.* **11**, 193–205.

World Health Organization (1958) *The First Ten Years of the World Health Organization.* WHO, Geneva.

World Health Organization (1993) *The Development of the WHO Quality of Life Assessment Instrument.* WHO, Geneva.

World Health Organization (2000) *General Guidelines for Methodologies on Research and Evaluation of Traditional Medicine.* WHO, Geneva (Foreword).

Zhang, J. and Wang, P. (2000) Quality of life and assessment of efficacy of Chinese medicine in cancer patients. *J. Beijing Univ. Tradit. Chin. Med.* **23**(2), 67–69.

Zhao, L. and Chan, K. (2003) Quality of life assessment: an outcome estimation of Chinese medical treatment. *Chin. J. Integr. Med.* **9**(4), 299–301.

Chapter 15

Clinical and Experimental Studies on Acupuncture-Drug Balanced Anaesthesia and Analgesia in China

Gen-cheng Wu

Abstract

The history of development of acupuncture anaesthesia was described. The application started with simple procedures like tooth extraction and eye operations, extending to neck operation, chest and abdominal operations. This incomplete analgesia has made the procedures imperfect. Since 1980, the direction of research has shifted to the combined use of acupuncture and anaesthetic drugs. Different studies have been completed. Acupuncture was used together with epidural anaesthesia, general anaesthesia and local anaesthesia. The advantages of the combined applications are discussed. Research to find out the mechanism of the synergistic effects is actively going on.

Keywords: Acupuncture; Anaesthesia; Analgesia.

15.1 Introduction

Acupuncture treatment is an important part of Traditional Chinese Medicine (TCM). For thousands of years, acupuncture has been proven effective in relieving pain. The ability of acupuncture to inhibit pain is referred as acupuncture analgesia. Since the establishment of the People's Republic of China in 1949, great progresses have been made in the research of acupuncture analgesia, guided by the principle of integration of Traditional Chinese and Western Medicine (Qian, 1986).

15.2 From Acupuncture Analgesia to Acupuncture Anaesthesia

Acupuncture anaesthesia was developed from acupuncture analgesia. The history of acupuncture anaesthesia can be traced back to as early as the 1950s (Zhang, 1989).

Originally, its discovery was prompted by the practice that stimulation of acupuncture points could relieve pain of the wound caused by the operation on the tonsil under local anaesthesia. Inspired by this experience, medical doctors tried to use acupuncture in tonsillectomy as a new anaesthetic measure in 1958. At that time, doctors of Chinese and Western medicine in the Shanghai First People's Hospital worked together and learnt from each other. They inserted needles into both sides of the Hegu (LI 4) point to relieve pain and the excellent result was showed repeatedly. After they believed that acupuncture could significantly increase the pain threshold and pain tolerance threshold, they applied it to actual tonsillectomy and achieved a satisfactory result. The first case of operation under acupuncture anaesthesia was performed on the 30 August 1958. Besides Shanghai, some medical doctors in other cities, such as Xián, Wuhan and Nanjing, finished other operations such as tooth extraction, operation for detachment of retina, thyroidectomy, appendectomy with acupuncture anaesthesia in the same or the following year (Zhang, 1989).

In 1960, the Shanghai First Tuberculosis Hospital and other hospitals in China succeeded in using acupuncture anaesthesia for pneumonectomy. After that, many other major and difficult operations (such as cardiac surgery, surgery on the anterior cranial fossa, total laryngectomy, subtotal gastrectomy, pan-hysterectomy, caesarean section, etc.) also got satisfactory results in the 1960s and 1970s (Zhang, 1989). However, in the beginning, the acupoints used for an operation generally were as many as dozens. This made it very inconvenient. Researchers in the Shanghai First Medical College (in 1985 the name was changed to the Shanghai Medical University, then in 2000 to the Shanghai Medical College, Fudan University) conducted observations on normal volunteers as well as patients, and found that the number of acupoints could be reduced markedly while the analgesic effect still remained the same, making it more feasible. On the other hand, the acupuncture was manipulated manually and the induction time was as long as 60 minutes at first. After some experiments, it was found that the manipulation of acupuncture could be managed by an electrical machine (electroacupuncture), and the induction time could be shortened to 20 minutes, with the same analgesic effect (Shanghai First Medical College, 1973).

More than 40 years have passed since the successful use of acupuncture anaesthesia in the first case. Substantial evidences have been accumulated that acupuncture has prominent analgesic effect and acupuncture anaesthesia is with scientific basis (Cao, 2002). It showed some advantages for surgical operation. However, because acupuncture plays its analgesic role via activating the endogenous pain modulating system, it fails to produce the complete abolishment of pain induced by surgical trauma (incomplete analgesia). This limitation hinders the wide use of acupuncture anaesthesia in clinic.

15.3 From Acupuncture Anaesthesia to Acupuncture-Drug Balanced Anaesthesia

Since the 1980s, the research of acupuncture anaesthesia has been continuing, although the cases of operation have decreased rapidly. Three national key projects supported by the Chinese central government were performed from 1986 to 2000. There were some famous hospitals, institutes and medical universities in Beijing, Shanghai, Chengdu and other cities joining in this national cooperation unit. The Shanghai Medical University had the honour of being appointed as the head of this unit (Wu and Cau, 1992; Cao, 1997; Wu *et al.*, 2001).

In recent years, the combination of acupuncture with drugs has been successfully used in anaesthesia for surgical operations such as open-heart surgery with cardiopulmonary bypass, pneumonectomy, craniocerebral operation, thyroidectomy, neolarynx reconstruction, subtotal gastrectomy, cholecystectomy, renal transplantation, etc. As previously known, in modern anaesthesiology, it is more common to use "balanced anaesthesia", in which various drugs and/or techniques cooperate with each other for an enhanced effect. Similarly, acupuncture can also play a cooperating role in combination with drugs, because it has an analgesic effect as well as a regulatory action on multiple important organs of the body, which usually cannot be substituted with drugs. Therefore, acupuncture combined with selected drugs to fulfill the requirement of anaesthesia is referred to as acupuncture-drug balanced anaesthesia, which can also be termed acupuncture balanced anaesthesia (Cao, 1997) or acupuncture assisted anaesthesia (Han, 1997).

The clinical application of acupuncture-drug balanced anaesthesia has its advantages: (1) acupuncture can be combined with different types of anaesthesia such as local anaesthesia, epidural anaesthesia and general anaesthesia, etc.; (2) the effect of analgesia was improved as the patients did not feel pain during the operation, and the post-operative pain was reduced as well; (3) the doses of analgesic or anaesthetic drugs were significantly decreased during the operation (usually by about one-third), hence side-effects were reduced; (4) the rate of the excellent effect of both operation and anaesthesia was increased; (5) many indexes of physiological condition became more stable; and (6) the post-operative recovery was accelerated, and the period of post-operative hospitalisation was shortened.

In the Affiliated Hospital of Chengdu University of TCM and Pharmacy, the clinical study on acupuncture combined with epidural administration of anaesthetics was reported in a total of 106 cases of cholecystectomy (Qin *et al.*, 2001). The patients were divided into group A, acupuncture + epidural; group B, acupoint-skin electrical stimulation + epidural; and group C, routine epidural. The excellent rate of these groups was 80%, 68.57% and 25%, respectively ($P < 0.001$). The surgeons and anaesthetists found some advantages in the combination of acupuncture with epidural anaesthesia: (1) the patients kept quiet; (2) the patients had no pain or only slight pain reaction; (3) muscular relaxation was satisfying; (4) the visceral-pulling reaction was light; (5) the dose of epidural anaesthetics required was decreased about 30%; and (6) the anaesthetic blocked level was markedly improved.

It was revealed that acupuncture and acupoint-skin electrical stimulation can reduce or suppress the stress response caused by surgical operation. Acupuncture can strengthen the analgesic effect of anaesthetics, lower the dose of epidural anaesthetics and raise lymphocyte-mediated immunocompetence.

Besides the cholecystectomy, the study of electroacupuncture combined with a low dose of epidural anaesthetic for subtotal gastrectomy was also reported in the same hospital (Qin *et al.*, 1996). It was concluded that electroacupuncture combined with a low dose of epidural anaesthetic is a method of anaesthesia to be considered for subtotal gastrectomy of benign pathological changes.

In the Sichuan Province Cancer Hospital, electroacupuncture combined with general anaesthesia for patients undergoing thoracic operation was observed in a total of 70 cases (Tang *et al.*, 2001). All patients were divided into group A, acupuncture + general anaesthesia; group B, acupoint-skin electrical stimulation + general/anaesthesia; and group C, general anaesthesia. The excellent rate of operation was 62.5%, 65.22% and 37.84%, respectively in these groups. It was found that the amount of anaesthetics in group A or B was reduced about 30%. The T-lymphocyte test indicated that acupuncture can up-regulate the immunofunction.

In the Renji Hospital Affiliated to Shanghai Second Medical University, the protective effect of electroacupuncture on patients undergoing cardiac surgery was investigated in 40 patients with atria septal defect (ASD) (Wang *et al.*, 2001). They were randomly allocated into three groups: group A, acupuncture + anaesthesia (12 cases); group B, acupuncture + general anaesthesia (12 cases); and group C, general anaesthesia (16 cases). Some haemodynamics parameters were observed in these cases, such as heart rate (HR), mean arterial pressure (MAP), cardiac output (CO), cardiac index (CI), stroke volume (SV) and systemic vascular resistance (SVR), etc. Several biochemical tests were analysed, such as superoxide dismutase (SOD), malonyldiadehyde (MDA) and creatine phosphokinase-isoenzyme (CPKI) extracted from blood samples of the internal jugular vein. Myocardial samples of the right auricle were taken for detection of the heat shock protein (HSP_{70}) mRNA expression. The results showed that acupuncture can adjust haemodynamics in patients undergoing cardiac operations, and enhance the ability of oxygen-derived free radical clearance and the expression of HSP_{70} mRNA. Acupuncture plus general anaesthesia may be the better method for reducing myocardial ischaemia-reperfusion injury.

In The Shanghai Lung Disease Hospital (the former Shanghai First Tuberculosis Hospital), a study on acupuncture anaesthesia for the operation of lung with vedio assistant thoracoscoy was carried out in 33 patients (Zhuo *et al.*, 2002). The result showed that the volume of the compound drug liquid used was in this group 43.5% less than that in the general anaesthesia group (33 cases, $P < 0.01$). They found that the blood pressure in the former group was more stable.

In the Huashan Hospital Affiliated to Shanghai Medical University, the clinical application of combined acupuncture-drug anaesthesia was reported in the cerebral functional area operation (Yan *et al.*, 1998). Satisfactory effects were obtained in all 80 patients, including 20 cases in the language center and 60 in the sensory and motor centers. The excellent rate of anaesthesia was 100%. After operation, no aggravation in dysphasia of dysfunction was found, and in the five cases, aggravation on myasthenia and dysesthesia was evident, but recovered within two to four weeks. The neurosurgery doctors find that the operation with combined acupuncture anaesthesia may result in high tumour resection rate and reduced incidence of disability. Therefore, this method of anaesthesia can be regarded as one of the routine anaesthesia methods.

In the Eye-Ear-Nose-Throat Hospital Affiliated to Shanghai Medical University, acupuncture anaesthesia combined with analgesics was performed in neoglottis reconstruction (Huang *et al.*, 2001). Thirty cases of glottic stenosis received laryngeal reconstruction under general anaesthesia. But after the operation, the lumen of the patients' larynxes was not large enough for respiration. So all the patients could not be decannulated. Then a new glottic reconstruction under combination of acupuncture with drugs was performed in these 30 patients, who maintained ideal consciousness and physiological states. Thus, the reconstructed new glottic easily achieved the physiological width. New glottic reconstruction under combination of acupuncture and local anaesthesia was performed by increasing the width of glottic lumen to about 4–5 mm. In this report, 28 cases were successfully decannulated with normal respiratory function, while only two cases failed in removing the tracheal cannula.

In the Shanghai First People's Hospital, the combined use of acupuncture with anaesthetics in renal transplantation can markedly reduce the consumption amounts of anaesthetics, which can improve the recovery of the transplanted renal functions and avoid complications (Qu *et al.*, 1996). It was found that the anaesthetic effect in patients under acupuncture-balanced anaesthesia was comparable to that under epidural block. The average amount of anaesthetics used in patients under acupuncture-balanced anaesthesia was only about half of that under epidural block.

The blood pressure and heart rate were stable during operation, and no hypertensor was needed in patients under acupuncture-balanced anaesthesia; while in patients under epidural block, the blood pressure often fluctuated. The start time of urination of transplanted kidney under acupuncture-balanced anaesthesia was significantly shortened compared with that under epidural block.

A further observation was performed in 44 case patients, which were divided into group A, routine dose of epidural block; group B, smaller dose of epidural block; groups C, routine dose of epidural block + electroacupuncture; and group D, smaller dose of epidural block + electroacupuncture (Wang *et al.*, 2002). It was found that electroacupuncture stimulation can really decrease the requirement of epidural anaesthetics, increase plasma epinephrine level, stabilise haemodynamics and improve the early renal function of the transplanted kidney under combined anaesthesia of electroacupuncture and epidural administration of small dose of anaesthetics.

15.4 Clinical and Experimental Research of Combination of Acupuncture with Drugs on Analgesia

In addition to the above examples of application of acupuncture combined with drugs in anaesthesia and surgical operations, the method of acupuncture combined with drugs can also be used in the treatment of analgesia, such as labour pain, back and leg pain, post-operative pain, etc.

In the Beijing Hospital for Gynecology and Obstetrics Affiliated to Beijing Capital Medical University, it was found that application of acupuncture stimulation with Han's acupoint nerve stimulator (HANS) combined with medicines was effective for pain relief during labour (Zhuang *et al.*, 2003). The results showed that the analgesic effective rate was 90.3% (group of HANS + diazepam) and 78.9% (group of HANS + tramadol), respectively. They were both higher than that in the group of HANS (59.8%, $p < 0.05$). HANS combined with a sedative or analgesic (diazepam and tramadol) had good analgesic effect on labour pain, and no side-effect was found in both mother and child. It was suggested that combination of HANS and diazepam or tramadol was safe, convenient and effective for relieving pain during labour.

In the Beijing Municipal TCM Hospital, the study of electroacupuncture combined with medicines for treatment of sciatica was reported in a total of 158 cases (Xu *et al.*, 2001). Five groups of patients were treated by the following methods: group A, electroacupuncture; group B, electroacupuncture + placebo; group C, electroacupuncture + nifedipine (calcium channel blocker); group D, electroacupuncture + beclofen (GABA receptor agonist); and group E, electroacupuncture + clonidine (alpha-2 receptor agonist of NA). The results showed that in partial patients, electroacupuncture has definite analgesic effect (28.00%). Electroacupuncture can improve the signs and strengthen locomotion. The drugs, such as clonidine and beclofen, can enhance the therapeutic effect of electroacupuncture, and the effective rate was 93.93% and 79.41% ($p < 0.001$).

In the Institute of Acupuncture and Moxibustion, Chinese Academy of TCM, the clinical study on analgesic effect of acupuncture and acupuncture combined with medicine was observed in post-operative pain of resection of nucleus pulposus of lumber intervertebral disc (Mo *et al.*, 2000).

Compared with the effect of dolantin, the analgesic effect of electroacupuncture initiated later, but remained longer. Therefore, the combination of acupuncture with a reduced dose of anaesthetics (dolantin) may be advisable. It was suggested that electroacupuncture should be applied earlier after operation to prevent pain occurrence, and a half-dose of dolantin may be used after acupuncture to achieve better analgesic effect.

In the Shanghai Medical University, the results of morphine combined with electroacupuncture were showed in the experimental and clinical studies (Dai *et al.*, 1993; Zhang and Cai, 1996). It is well known that epidural morphine is commonly used in clinic to relieve post-operative pains, but at the same time it induces immuno-suppression, inhibition of the intestinal peristalsis and respiratory inhibition. The results of our research group indicated that when morphine was combined with electroacupuncture, side-effects induced by morphine became mild.

15.5 Mechanism of Synergistic Effect of Acupuncture-Drug Combination

Using animal models, we screened some commonly used clinical drugs in our laboratory (Xu *et al.*, 1989). They can be classified into three main categories (according to their effect on acupuncture analgesia): (1) drugs with potentiating effect; (2) drugs with reducing effect, and (3) drugs without significant influence. It provides the clinical principles for medical doctors to select the proper adjuvant based on different conditions.

For drugs with potentiating effect, their pharmacological types are divided into: (1) agonists of opioid receptors — fentanyl and pethidine; (2) antagonists of dopamine (DA) receptors — droperidol, haloperido, clozapine, rotundine, perphenazine, 1-stepholikine tetrahydroprotoberbine, domperidone and SCH 23390; (3) serotonin (5-HT) release — fenfluramine; and (4) drugs affecting the multiple functions — metoclopramide (clinically used as an anti-emetic, with actions of anti-cholinesterase and anti-dopamine) and tetrahydrocannabinol (can bind to the μ-opioid receptor and inhibit the synthesis of DA and norepinephrine, NE).

In recent years, the mechanism of some drugs affecting acupuncture analgesia has been investigated by using multi-disciplinary techniques (Zhu *et al.*, 1997).

Endogenous opioid peptides (EOP) play an important role in inhibiting pain (He, 1987). It has been known that EOP release is increased during analgesia. Further work showed that EOP release was promoted by the combination of acupuncture with potentiating drugs. Electroacupuncture induced increase not only in affinity but also in the density of the opioid receptors, and the combined use of acupuncture with drugs further enhanced this increase, suggesting that further activation of the opioid receptors may underlie the mechanism of the drugs' potentiating effect on acupuncture analgesia. These drugs can also play their potentiating role in acupuncture-induced activity of EOP gene expression.

Besides EOP, monoamine transmitters including DA, NE and 5-HT, play different roles in acupuncture analgesia. Using techniques of *in vivo* microdialysis and high performance liquid chromatography with electrochemical detection (HPLC-ECD), the monoamine contents in microdialysate from rat brain areas were measured before and after some drugs enhanced electroacupuncture analgesia. The results suggested that these drugs potentiated acupuncture analgesia not only via antagonising the activity of dopaminergic system, but coordinating the activities of other monoamine such as 5-HT in the brain (Li *et al.*, 1999).

The Beijing Medical University and the Shanghai Medical University are two of the most prestigious research groups focusing on the relationship between EOP and acupuncture. In 1995, orphanin FQ (also named nociceptin, OFQ), a newly discovered member of the opioid family, was found. They observed that this opioid peptide was also involved in acupuncture analgesia, but showed different effects in the brain or spinal cord. It was found that OFQ had an antagonistic action on acupuncture analgesia in the brain (Zhu *et al.*, 1996; Tian *et al.*, 1997), but in the spinal cord, the enhancing effect of OFQ on acupuncture analgesia was significant (Tian *et al.*, 1997). In OFQ knockout mice, the analgesic effect induced by electroacupuncture at 100 Hz was significantly stronger (You *et al.*, 2001). It was suggested that endogenous OFQ appeared to increase the sensitivity of nociception and played an antagonistic role in 100 Hz electroacupuncture analgesia.

Endomorphine, the endogenous ligand of the μ-receptor, was discovered in 1997. It was showed that endomorphin-1 mediated 2 Hz but not 100 Hz electroacupuncture analgesia in the rats (Han *et al.*, 1999). Another result showed that OFQ at the supraspinal level produced hyperalgesia and was antagonistic to endomorphin-1, while at the spinal level it produced analgesia and was synergic with endomorphin-1 (Wang *et al.*, 1999).

On the other hand, the analgesic effect can be found in some biologically active substances, such as melatonin (Yu *et al.*, 2000). That effect related with the EOP system was also investigated. Melatonin can enhance acupuncture analgesia involved in the EOP system, suggesting potential clinical application as an assisted analgesic in the near future (Zhou *et al.*, 2000; 2001).

References

Cao, X. (1997) From acupuncture anaesthesia to acupuncture balanced anaesthesia. *World J. Acupunct. Mox.* **7**(4), 19–24.

Cao, X. (2002) Scientific bases of acupuncture analgesia. *Acupunct. Electrother. Res. Int. J.* **27**, 1–14.

Dai, J., Ren, Z., Fu, Z. and Zhu, Y. (1993) Electroacupuncture reversed the inhibition of intestinal peristalsis induced by intrathecal injection of morphine in rabbits. *Chin. Med. J.* **106**(3), 220–224.

Department of Physiology, Shanghai First Medical College, Shanghai First Tuberculosis Hospital and Shanghai Institute of Acupuncture and Moxibustion (1973) *Effect of Acupuncture of Points on the Pain Threshold of Normal Human Subjects.* Selection of Research on Acupuncture Anaesthesia, Shanghai People' Press, pp. 33–39 (in Chinese).

Han, J. (1997) Acupuncture anaesthesia versus acupuncture-assisted anaesthesia. *World J. Acupunct. Mox.* **7**(4), 16–18.

Han, Z., Jiang, Y., Wan, Y., Wang, Y., Chang, J. and Han J. (1999) Endomorphin-1 mediates 2 Hz but not 100 Hz electroacupuncture analgesia in the rats. *Neurosci. Lett.* **274**(2), 75–78.

He, L. (1987) Involvement of endogenous opioid peptides in acupuncture analgesia. *Pain* **31**, 99–121.

Huang, H., Tian, X., Zhou, C., Zhou, A. and Shao, Q. (2001) Application of acupuncture anaesthesia combined with analgesics to neoglottis reconstruction. *Acupunct. Res.* **26**(1), 35–37 (in Chinese with English abstract).

Li, X., Zhu, C., Chen, H., Zhu, Y., Wu, G. and Xu, S. (1999) Effects of fenfluramine combined with electroacupuncture on monoamine release in periaqueductal gray of rat brain. *Acta Pharmacol. Sin.* **20**(7), 597–600.

Mo, X., Chen, Z. and Shi, H. (2000) A clinical study on analgesic effect of acupuncture and acupuncture combined with medicine on postoperative pain of resection of nucleus pulposus of lumber intervertebral disc. *Acupunct. Res.* **25**(4), 296–299 (in Chinese with English abstract).

Qian, X. (1986) Progress in scientific research on acupuncture, moxibustion and acupuncture analgesia by integrating traditional Chinese and Western medicine. In: *Research on Acupuncture, Moxibustion and Acupuncture Anaesthesia*, (ed.) Zhang, X., Science Press, Beijing, 1986, pp. 1–18.

Qin, B., Liu, Y., Cheng, X., Peng, Q., Sun, Y., Chen, W. and Zhang, L. (1996) Electroacupuncture combined with low dose epidural anaesthesia for subtotal gastrectomy. *Chin. J. Pain Med.* **2**(3), 135–143 (in Chinese with English abstract).

Qin, B., Ren, Y., Zhang, L., Bai, Z., Hu, B., Yin, D., Yang, J. and Wang, D. (2001) Summary of the clinical study on acupuncture combined with epidural injection of small dose of anaesthetic for cholecystectomy. *Acupunct. Res.* **26**(2), 143–149 (in Chinese with English abstract).

Qu, G., Zhuang, X., Xu, G., Yang, L., Wang, Z., Chen, S., Wang, S., Xu, D. and Xie, T. (1996) Clinical observation on combined anaesthetics acupuncture anaesthesia in 50 patients undergoing renal transplantation. *Chin. J. Pain Med.* **2**(2), 72–77 (in Chinese with English abstract).

Tang, Y., Qin, B., Hu, B., Wei, X. and Yin, Z. (2001) Clinical study on the effect of acupuncture combined with enflurane general anaesthesia for esophagectomy. *Acupunct. Res.* **26**(2), 138–142 (in Chinese with English abstract).

Tian, J., Xu, W., Zhang, W., Fang, Y., Grisel, J.E., Mogil, J., Grandy, S., David, K. and Han, J. (1997) Involvement of endogenous orphanin FQ in electroacupuncture-induced analgesia. *NeuroReport* **8**, 497–500.

Wan, Y., Peng, B., Pintar, J.E. and Han, J. (2001) Potentiation of electro-acupuncture analgesia in orphnin FQ knockout mice. *Chin. J. Pain Med.* **7**(3), 161–164 (in Chinese with English abstract).

Wang, X., Lu, Z., Xu, C., Hang, Y. and Sun, D. (2001) The protective effects of electroacupuncture on patients undergoing cardiac surgery. *Acupunct. Res.* **26**(3), 173–174 (in Chinese with English abstract).

Wang, Y., Zhu, C., Wu, G., Cao, X., Wang, Y. and Cui, D. (1999) Effects of orphanin FQ endomorphine-1 induced analgesia. *Brain Res.* **835**, 241–246.

Wang, Z., Li, S., Zhuang, X., Ma, H., Xu, G., Wang, Z., Chen, S., Tao, A. and Xu, D. (2002) Effect of acupuncture combined with epidural anaesthesia on early function of transplanted kidney. *Chin. Acupunct. Mox.* **22**(9), 613–616 (in Chinese with English abstract).

Wu, G. and Cao, X. (1992) Recent achievements in acupuncture anaesthesia in China, *World J. Acupunct. Mox.* **2**(3), 39–42.

Wu, G., Chen, Z. and Qin, B. (2001) Improvement of anaesthesia and analgesia of acupuncture combined with drugs: clinical observation and experimental research. *Acupunct. Res.* **26**(3), 161–162 (in Chinese with English abstract).

Xu, J., Liu, J., Zhang, Y., Zhang, D., Li, Y. and Fang, Z. (2001) Electroacupuncture combined with medicines for treatment of sciatica. *Acupunct. Res.* **26**(3), 187–188 (in Chinese with English abstract).

Xu, S., Cao, X., Mo, W., Xu, Z. and Pan, Y. (1989) Effect of combination of drugs with acupuncture analgesic efficacy. *Acupunct. Electrother. Res. Int. J.* **4**, 103–113.

Yan, H., Jiang, C. and Liang, W. (1998) Clinical application of combined acupuncture-drug anaesthesia in cerebral functional area operation. *Chin. J. Integr. Tradit. West. Med.* **18**(3), 138–139 (in Chinese with English abstract).

Yu, C., Zhu, C., Xu, S., Cao, X. and Wu, G. (2000) The analgesic effects of peripheral and central administration of melatonin in rats. *Eur. J. Pharmacol.* **403**, 49–53.

Zhang, R. (1989) *Developmental History of Acupuncture Anaesthesia in China.* Shanghai Scientific and Technical Literature Publisher, Shanghai, 1989, pp. 8–32 (in Chinese).

Zhang, Y. and Cao, X. (1996) Electroacupuncture (EA)-induced attenuation of immunosuppression appearing after epidural or intrathecal injection of morphine in patients and rats. *Acupunct. Electrother. Res. Int. J.* **21**, 177–186.

Zhou, H., Dong, W., Liu, S. and Zhang, M. (2002) Study on acupuncture anaesthesia for the operation of lung with vedio assistant thoracoscoy. *Acupunct. Res.* **22**(2), 105–107 (in Chinese with English abstract).

Zhou, M., Yu, C., Cao, X. and Wu, G. (2001) Alteration of Oorphanin FQ immunoreactivity and ppOFQ mRNA by combination of melatonin with electroacupuncture. *Acupunct. Electrother. Res. Int. J.* **26**, 49–58.

Zhou, M., Yu, C., Cao, X. and Wu, G. (2002) Effects of melatonin on electro-acupuncture analgesia in rats. *Acupunct. Res.* **25**(2), 93–95 (in Chinese with English abstract).

Zhu, C., Xu, S., Cao, X., *et al.* (1996) Antagonistic actions orphanin FQ on acupuncture analgesia in rat brain. *Acupunct. Electrother. Res.* **21**, 199–205.

Zhu, C., Xu, S., Wu, G. and Cao, X. (1997) Research on combination of acupuncture with drugs. *World J. Acupunct. Mox.* **7**(4), 54–59.

Zhuang, S., Wu, L., Fan, L., Jin, Y., Lui, W., Han, X., Hu, T., Wang, Y., Tian, C., Liu, Y. and Zhao, T. (2003) Combination of acupuncture and drugs for pain relief during labour. *Chin. J. Perinat. Med.* **6**(1), 6–9 (in Chinese with English abstract).

Chapter 16

Approaches in Developing an Integrative and Evidence-Based Curriculum in Chinese Herbal Medicine

Kylie A. O'Brien, Robyn Lines & Charlie C.L. Xue

Abstract

In Australia, Chinese medicine is practiced within a complex health care system in which western medicine is dominant. Chinese medicine is an evolving medical system in terms of practice and education, and has moved into western settings. For Chinese medicine to develop in western countries there needs to be integration of Chinese medicine with western medicine, not only from the point of knowledge about the human state of existence but in the sense of integration of Chinese medicine within the context of a western health care system that is built around western medicine, the dominant form of health care within western countries. It is important that educational programmes in Chinese medicine are not only consistent with the philosophy of Chinese medicine but are relevant to the context in which Chinese medicine is practiced.

In the development of RMIT University's Master of Applied Science (Chinese Herbal Medicine), an educational approach was adopted that emphasises the integration of western medicine and Chinese medicine. Chinese medicine is beginning to be studied using the same scientific research methodology that is applied to western medicine and that increasingly is used to guide clinical practice. The evidence-based approach to the study and practice of Chinese herbal medicine has been adopted in the curriculum development and implementation. This is an illustration of the bridging process that is beginning to occur in both China and as Chinese medicine establishes itself within western settings.

The overall programme design was guided by a *capability-based* approach, one in which the holistic capability that is the desired outcome of the study programme is identified and used to guide all aspects of the curriculum design. A "capability map" was constructed. The first step was identification of four dimensions of capabilities needed to achieve an overall capability of being able to practice Chinese herbal medicine in a professional manner. Necessary skills and abilities needed to achieve the capabilities and underpinning these skills, the enabling knowledge, were defined. The capabilities, skills and abilities and enabling knowledge were then mapped over individual courses (subjects) within the programme. The integration of western medicine and Chinese medicine occurred at each of the levels of the capability map, i.e. at the level of specific capabilities, underpinning skills and abilities and enabling knowledge, and was applied within courses across the programme. This paper illustrates ways in which an integrative and evidence based approach was used to develop an innovative Chinese herbal medicine curriculum in which Chinese medicine and western medicine are integrated.

Keywords: Capability-Based Curriculum; Integration; Evidence Based Medicine; Chinese Herbal Medicine Education.

16.1 Introduction

In the development of Chinese medicine curricula, it is important to consider the changing context within which Chinese medicine is practised so that graduates are able to integrate as practitioners within the health care system now and adapt to changing professional contexts in the future. An approach that integrates knowledge of Chinese and western medicine is necessary if Chinese medicine is to continue to develop as a medicine in the 21st century. An evidence-based approach to Chinese medicine in which practitioners consider clinical issues armed with an understanding of what evidence is and how it can guide practice will further contribute to the development of clinical practice and may eventually facilitate the move of Chinese medicine into mainstream health care in western countries like Australia.

The Royal Melbourne Institute of Technology (RMIT) University in Melbourne, Australia, has developed a new Masters degree programme that features an integrated and evidence-based curriculum in Chinese herbal medicine and aims to equip graduates with the capabilities to practise within the Australian health care system and within future professional contexts. One of the key features of this programme is the integration of

Chinese and western medicine, not only in terms of integration of knowledge from both systems about the human state of existence but in terms of integration of Chinese medicine within a western health care setting that is based around western medicine. The programme design used a *capability-based* approach to curriculum development.

This paper will discuss the factors taken into consideration in the curriculum design, the features of the curriculum and how a capability-based approach was used to create an integrative and innovative curriculum in Chinese herbal medicine.

16.2 Factors of Consideration in the Design of a Chinese Medicine Curriculum

A number of factors were taken into consideration in the design of the Chinese herbal medicine curriculum. These include the context of Chinese medicine practice in Australia, the integration of Chinese and western medicine that is occurring and needs to occur, evaluation of quality of health care including the shift towards an evidence-based practice, and the kinds of capabilities needed by graduates in order to practice professionally, adapt to changing professional contexts and continue life-long learning.

16.2.1 *The context of Chinese medicine practice in Australia*

Chinese medicine is relatively new to western countries and is becoming an increasingly popular form of health care. In Australia, Chinese medicine is practised within a complex health care system in which western medicine is dominant, and it is practised predominantly within private practice. In addition, an estimated 15% of Australian general practitioners also practice acupuncture (Easthope *et al.*, 1998), and acupuncture practised by western medical practitioners is rebatable under Australia's Medicare system (though not if practised by a Chinese medicine practitioner who is not also a western medical practitioner). "Medical acupuncture" that is often practised by western medical practitioners is not the same as traditional acupuncture guided by Chinese medicine theory. In contrast, in China and Vietnam, Chinese medicine is practised predominantly in hospitals and is well integrated with western medicine within the health care system. In China there are both Chinese and western medicine hospitals, and within the Chinese medicine hospitals, western medical diagnostic facilities are available and utilised. Chinese medicine doctors may prescribe western medication if indicated. Acupuncture has begun to be practised in a limited way within a few Australian hospitals.

The context within which Chinese medicine is practised within Australia is one that is changing and becoming increasingly regulated. The state of Victoria was the first state in a western country to regulate the practice of Chinese medicine and other states/territories may follow suit. Professional associations also provide a form of self-regulation within Australia's states and territories. Proprietary forms of Chinese medicines are regulated by the Commonwealth government's Therapeutic Goods Administration. Raw herbs are more loosely regulated, though certain toxic herbs are subject to state/territory drugs and poisons legislation. Private health insurance companies have recognised the popularity of Chinese medicine with an increasing number of companies now providing rebates for acupuncture and Chinese herbal medicine treatments. Chinese medicine is also becoming increasingly regulated in other parts of the world including China and Europe.

Chinese medicine is a developing profession within Australia and other western countries. Chinese medicine needs to embrace a similar level of professionalism as western medicinc if it is to gain credibility within the Australia health care system and if it is to eventually move into mainstream health care. Chinese medicine curricula therefore have to develop in graduates an appreciation of professionalism including ethics and an understanding of the regulations that govern provision of Chinese medicine services within Australia.

Chinese medicine education has entered mainstream education institutions and universities. RMIT University was the first university in Australia to develop a five-year double degree undergraduate programme in Chinese medicine and human biology teaching both main modalities of Chinese medicine: acupuncture and Chinese herbal medicine. A number of other Australian universities have also developed four- and five-year degree programmes.

The context of practice of Chinese medicine has changed markedly on a global level. Chinese medicine practice and education has moved outside of China and other Asian countries and into western countries. Tremendous changes have occurred within Australia over the past 15 years. It is important that Chinese medicine curricula equip graduates with not only the capabilities to be able to practice within the current professional contexts but to be able to practice within future professional contexts that may be quite different to those of today.

16.2.2 *Integration of Chinese and western medicine*

Integration of Chinese and western medicine is occurring now, in particular because of the context in which it is practised. Education needs to recognise this contextual driver that includes how our health care system is set up (around western medicine) and cultural changes in western medicine that are and will impact on Chinese medicine, specifically the shift towards evidence-based practice. At another level, integration has the potential to contribute profoundly to our understanding of the human state of existence, health and illness.

The Australian health care system is established to (predominantly) support the western model of health care that is based on a biomedical understanding of disease and treatment. Chinese medicine, being a relatively new health care means, has limited option but to integrate into the western health care system. Professionalism and rigour in clinical practice is being demanded in Chinese medicine commensurate with what is demanded in western medicine. This is illustrated by the various practice guidelines that are being developed by the Chinese Medicine Registration Board of Victoria and professional associations representing Chinese medicine practitioners (for example, provision of infection control guidelines for acupuncture) and by provision of systems to deal with unprofessional conduct and complaints against practitioners. That is not to say that Chinese medicine did not have its own sense of professionalism historically, but simply to suggest that the structures that have been and are being put into place within Australia are reflective of a western health care model that is based on western medicine. Chinese medicine practitioners in Victoria, for example, must have professional indemnity insurance in order to gain and maintain registration: this need for protection against potential litigation is another by-product of the western health care setting.

Chinese medicine practitioners are bound by certain pieces of legislation. This applies not only to practitioners in the state of Victoria where there is statutory regulation of Chinese medicine, but within other states and territories. For example, state and territory drugs and poisons legislation impact on access to raw herbs that are considered toxic, and other state and territory legislation impact on acupuncturists via requirements for infection control. There are other examples of integration of Chinese medicine into a western health care system.

Historically there is evidence that the integration of western and Chinese medicine knowledge is not new: exchanges of knowledge between the Chinese and Europeans have been occurring for centuries (Cai *et al.*, 1995; Cheng, 1987). With the arrival of western missionaries in the 19th century, western medicine began to spread throughout China and in the 20th century, became established as a system of medicine that exists side by side with Chinese medicine (Cai *et al.*, 1995). However, integration of Chinese and western medicine had begun before the time of occupation of China by various European countries in the 19th and early 20th centuries. For example, at the end of the 17th century, a text entitled *The Origin of Medicine* was written that focused on the integration of Chinese and western medicine (Cai *et al.*, 1995), and in 1899 the book *Illustration of the Bronze Figure with Chinese and Western Medicine* was written that facilitated the approach of studying acupuncture using a combination of western and Chinese medicine (Cheng, 1987). In modern times, during the 20th century, the Communist Party encouraged the cooperation between western and Chinese medicine (Cai *et al.*, 1995). In China, Chinese medicine education entered universities in the 20th century, and western medical knowledge forms a substantial part of Chinese medical training. Similarly, students training in western medicine are required to complete some training in Chinese medicine.

Notwithstanding the fact that Chinese medicine has a fundamentally different understanding of the human state of existence and the aetiology and pathogenesis of disease than western medicine, and that this understanding is couched in terms of Chinese medicine theory, Chinese and western medicines have continued to integrate in terms of identification and understanding of diseases. In Chinese medicine, each disease or disorder typically has between three and five diagnostic sub-categories called "syndromes". Each syndrome is characterised by typical signs and symptoms that are reflective of the underlying aetiology and pathology, according to Chinese theory, and treatment is specific for the syndrome identified. In more modern times, knowledge has emerged about a range of conditions according to western medical understanding, for example, irritable bowel syndrome, benign prostatic hyperplasia and hypercholesterolaemia. In past centuries, Chinese medicine may have treated the chief presenting signs and/or symptoms and the understanding of aetiology and pathogenesis was couched in terms of Chinese medicine theory, no less logical than western medical theory, simply different. However, there has been a shift towards integration in terms of identifying disease according to western medicine (that may require the use of western medical diagnostic tests) and applying the theory of Chinese medicine to the understanding of aetiology, pathogenesis and treatment of such modern diseases, including the sub-categorisation of diseases into various diagnostic sub-categories or syndromes.

Integration of Chinese and western medicine in terms of treatment is also occurring. Chinese medicine may also be used to support western medical treatment. For example, acupuncture and/or herbal medicine may help alleviate side effects of chemotherapy in cancer patients. And the increase in western medical practitioners and allied health practitioners such as chiropractors, osteopaths and physiotherapists who are using acupuncture in their practices is just another example of how Chinese and western medicine are integrating.

Western and Chinese medicine have begun to integrate in terms of understanding the pharmacological actions on the body of various herbs and herbal medicine categories. For example, many of the herbs in the "dampness draining herbs" category are diuretics and many of the herbs in the "clear heat and relieve toxicity" category have anti-inflammatory and anti-pyretic actions (Bensky and Gamble, 1993). The neurological basis of acupuncture has been studied widely and the neuronal pathways of acupuncture analgesia have been described using various models, the most well-known theory being the "Gate Theory". Certain Chinese herbs have formed the basis for promising western drugs, for example, the extract Artemisinin from the herb Qing Hao is a promising anti-malarial drug, and Ephedrine is extracted from the herb Ma Huang (Tang and Wong, 1998).

Chinese medicine has, as its basis, an understanding of the human body that is described in terms of energy (termed qi) and inter-dependent organ systems and recognises the inter-dependence of man and the environment. This view is fundamentally different from the understanding of the body according to western medicine. Such differences in approaches to understanding the human state of existence boil down to differences in paradigms that will eventually need to be addressed if western and Chinese medicine are to truly integrate. This is work for the future. The bridging of understanding between western and Chinese medicines is the only logical step forward in the development of Chinese medicine in the future. Both systems of medicines have knowledge to bring to the other about understanding how humans function as multi-dimensional beings, how disease occurs and how health may be improved.

At a very practical level, Chinese medicine practitioners need to be able to understand the nature of the body and disease according to the (western) biomedical paradigm in order to work within a health system that is dominated by western medicine. In order for many diseases to be diagnosed, Chinese medicine practitioners may need to refer to western medical practitioners. In Australia, certain western medical diagnostic tests such as pathology tests, radiology reports and biopsies cannot be ordered by Chinese medicine practitioners: Chinese medicine practitioners need to be able to liaise with medical practitioners and need to be proficient in western medical language. There is no point in trying to talk to a general practitioner about "damp-heat in the lower jiao" *instead of* the western medical term "urinary tract infection" when the western medical practitioner does not understand Chinese medicine theory or terminology. In addition, there are medico-legal aspects to consider in the treatment with Chinese medicine of patients who may have serious illness that is and/or remains undiagnosed.

For all of the afore-mentioned reasons, Chinese medicine curricula need to integrate Chinese and western medicine.

16.2.3 *Evidence-based medicine*

Evidence-based medicine (EBM) has become popular in relatively recent times in western medicine and increasingly guides clinical practice. Sackett and colleagues provide a useful definition of EBM: "Evidence-based medicine is the conscientious, explicit and judicious use of current best evidence in making decisions about the case of individual patients. The practice of evidence-based medicine means integrating individual clinical expertise with the best available clinical evidence from systematic research" (Sackett *et al.*, 1996: p. 1). Systematic scientific evidence comes in many forms including randomised clinical trials, meta-analyses, cross-sectional studies, individual case studies and basic (laboratory) research. Rosenberg describes EBM as "an approach to clinical problem solving, a means of determining rational practice, a method of integrating service with training and education, a way of generating research ideas and, in summary, best practice made explicit and accessible" (Rosenberg, 2001: p. 1). It may also be a way in which to resolve health economic issues through elimination of practises that are not effective (Rosenberg, 2001). If Chinese medicine is to become accepted by the western medical community, it will need to be scrutinised in the same way that western medicine is.

There are many reasons for applying the EBM approach to Chinese medicine. It is not for the purpose of justifying itself to the western medicine fraternity, though this may well be an effect: it is to explore the medicine in as many ways as possible in order to understand and develop Chinese medicine further. Chinese medicine is not flawless nor has it reached its full potential. Development of an evidence base to which scientific research contributes will not only help guide clinical practice, but may also help bridge the understanding of the human including health and illness between western and Chinese medicine.

Putting Chinese medicine under the microscope and studying it according to the best scientific principles can produce useful information that can help guide clinical practice and provide a level of justification for particular clinical treatments, including the prescription of particular herbal medicines and acupuncture prescriptions. Research may provide a scientific basis for further development of Chinese medicine theory (Tang and Wong, 1998). Chinese medicine treatments shown to be effective through well-designed research may identify future directions of laboratory research, for example inquiry into mechanisms of action, in fields of pharmacology, physiology and biochemistry (Tang and Wong, 1998). Chinese medicine has provided the basis of some very successful orthodox drugs and this should not be seen as threatening to the integrity of Chinese medicine. Instead, it is an example of integration.

Chinese medicine does not, however, readily lend itself to a reductionist approach that often characterises western scientific research. Clinical studies need to be well designed and take into account the underlying theories and principles that guide Chinese medicine, otherwise results may not be clinically useful. At the very least, research into Chinese medicine that does not take this into account needs to admit potential limitations when making conclusions about results of research.

Research results need to reach practitioners, and practitioners need to be able to understand the scientific research methodology and language in order to be able to critically evaluate research. At a fundamental level, practitioners need to develop a mindset that demands to know what evidence there is that something works and by which criteria can this be judged so. In order to do so, Chinese medicine practitioners need to be equipped with the skills and knowledge in basic biostatistics and epidemiological research methodology and understand the many complexities of research into Chinese medicine. Training should also include how to use databases and conduct a strategic search of and critically appraise the literature (Richardson, 2002). In the design of Chinese medicine curricula, it is therefore important to integrate an evidence-based approach to the study of Chinese medicine as well as specifically provide opportunities to learn the afore-mentioned skills. This is another example of integration of Chinese medicine with western medicine.

16.3 Design of a Chinese Herbal Medicine Curriculum

The aim of the curriculum ultimately is to provide the framework for a Chinese medicine programme in which graduates can develop the capabilities necessary to practise in a professional manner within not only the current professional context but also within future professional contexts that may be different to those today.

The programme has been tailored for students within a western health care setting: one of the explicit aims of the course is that students will demonstrate capabilities at a practitioner level in relation to the health care system in Australia and internationally.

Some of the key elements of the curriculum were:

(1) Grounding of the programme in the context of practice: within a western health care setting, including the inter-leaving of ethics and regulatory frameworks throughout the programme.
(2) Integration of Chinese and western medicine. This was achieved via presentation of medical knowledge from both Chinese and western medicine viewpoints, particularly within the clinical courses, and the integration of an evidence-based approach to the study, practice and research of Chinese medicine throughout the programme.

An educational approach was adopted in the development of the curriculum that was both innovative and integrative in order to achieve the desired objectives of the programme. The approach was a *capability-based approach* to curriculum development. The educational philosophy behind the capability-based approach and features of the curriculum model will be discussed in the following section. The remainder of the paper will discuss the actual development of a capability-based curriculum for the Master of Applied Science (Chinese Herbal Medicine) at RMIT University, and will illustrate the inherent integrative nature of the approach: in particular, how it facilitates integration of Chinese and western medicine including the development of an evidence-based approach throughout the programme.

16.3.1 *Educational philosophy and approach*

A capability-based approach to curriculum development was one in which the holistic and integrated capability that is the desired outcome of the programme of study is defined and used to guide all aspects of curriculum design from broad curriculum structure to the detailed design of component courses. The approach is very integrative by nature.

The concept of capability that underpins the approach is different from previous curriculum concerns that have emphasised the development of generic skills. Past approaches have focussed on development of discipline or content knowledge (i.e. the ability to talk about areas of knowledge) and the development of skills often occurred in isolation from and as additions to discipline knowledge. Discipline knowledge plus learning of skills does not necessarily produce capability to practise in the case of a primary health care professional. In a capability-based approach, discipline and professional knowledge and skills are understood as a means to an end. The end that is desired includes but goes beyond the ability to practice effectively in current professional contexts. It is predicated on the understanding that in times of rapid change, graduates will practice in radically different professional worlds from those we currently know. According to this view, university students need to be prepared for a future that is largely unknown. Traditionally acquired discipline knowledge will not be enough to enable them to effectively negotiate situations that they have never before encountered. Rather they will require the ability to critically evaluate novel situations, determine what is salient in them, design and implement solutions drawing upon both disciple knowledge and broad capabilities in such domains as communication and information management. What becomes essential is the ability to continuously re-negotiate meaning and practice in a turbulent world and through this to continue to build understanding (Bowden *et al.*, 2000). To achieve such a capability, discipline knowledge and skills need to be integrated.

The emphasis is on a holistic or integrated notion of capability and such approaches have gained increasing support. Stephenson (1995: p. 24) defined capability as, "having justified confidence in your ability to (1) take appropriate and effective action, (2) communicate effectively, (3) collaborate with others, and (4) learn from experience, within familiar and unfamiliar circumstances". A recent Business and Higher Education Round Table (BHERT) paper (2003: pp. 9 and 12) described capability as, "growing understanding of how to deal with different contexts" and even more broadly, "a reflection of the kind of person one is". This form of holistic capability has been contrasted with the outcomes of traditional educational approaches that have been widely criticised as failing to produce graduates who can perform adequately in practice (see for example Industry Task Force on Leadership and Management Skills, 1995; A C Nielsen Research Services, 2000; Harvey, 2000).

General statements of holistic capability such as those quoted above are necessarily vague and the first stage of any capability-based curriculum development must be an understanding of holistic capability that is specific to the outcomes of the particular area of study and the discipline or professional practice for which it is a preparation. The grounding of a statement of capability for a specific domain of education can usefully draw upon consultations with interested stakeholders from industry, the community, other academics and learners. For the Chinese herbal medicine Masters degree, extensive use was made of documents generated by professional and regulatory bodies and dialogue with current practitioners, educators, students and alumni.

The idea of starting with an explicit statement of the desired integrated outcome from a programme of study challenges traditional curriculum approaches. It requires a transformation of practice from design strategies that most often arrive at a curriculum by a process of accumulation from discrete courses that are developed and "owned" by individual academics. The development of a profile of the desired holistic capability, on the contrary, provides a reference point for the design of curriculum structures and individual courses so that the focus remains on the achievement of capability and does not become limited to the acquisition of discipline knowledge or discrete skills. In a capability-based approach, learning outcomes are still used to describe the purposes of specific courses. These outcomes are, however, predominantly performative and are articulated in relation to the broader capability they underpin. In the case of Chinese medicine, the holistic capability identified rested upon an understanding of the dual nature of integration in this domain. At the level of content and practice, there is the need to integrate Western medicine and Chinese medicine traditions in theory and practice. At the curriculum design level there is the need to integrate all learning so that a holistic capability results that provides the basis for continuing practice and practice development in the dynamic and unpredictable social and political environment that the continuing development of Chinese medicine in a western health care environment ensures.

The development of capability is underpinned by a particular learning theory. It is consistent with a constructivist approach, as students must be active in constructing meaning, critically evaluating their developing capability and shaping their learning experiences. Variation theory (Bowden and Marton, 1998), in particular, provides the learning framework at RMIT University. Variation theory argues that developing the capability to discern relevant aspects in a situation comes from experiencing variation in situations and contexts so that similarities and differences are perceived and ways of identifying the most salient features of a novel situation are developed. The key is not just in having varied experiences but also actually experiencing the variation, which requires that it be the subject of reflection and analysis. Without this reflective, analytic activity varied experiences in themselves are insufficient to develop capability (*Ibid*, p. 154). The theory also suggests that the more the situations dealt with by students resemble the complexity and multi-factorial nature of real life, the more likely that a robust and effective capability will be developed.

The concept of holistic capability when combined with an understanding of variation theory for learning suggests a range of approaches for curriculum structure, teaching and assessment. A capability-based curriculum must provide space for students to develop, practise and demonstrate their ability to integrate knowledge and specific aspects of the overall capability learned in separate courses and contexts so that they can address significant, novel and messy, "real world" problems and professional practice situations. This can take many curriculum forms that include work-integrated learning streams, clinical practicums, studio courses and problem- or research-based capstone courses.

A capability-based curriculum must also provide opportunities for students to become critically aware of their developing capability. Approaches to this dimension of curriculum include learning portfolios, hurdle assessments of capability and self and peer assessments.

16.4 Development of a Capability-Based Curriculum

The programme design began with identifying an overall capability. This was simply expressed as *being able to practise Chinese herbal medicine in a professional manner* but was understood within the broader context

Table 16.1. Four dimensions of the overall capability and examples.

Dimension of overall capability	Example
Technical capabilities	The ability to formulate a herbal prescription or make modifications to formulae based on an understanding of the components, indications and contraindications of a number of commonly used herbs and Chinese herbal formulae
Communication capabilities	The ability to communicate (bilaterally) effectively with patients, other health professionals, regulatory bodies, herbal uppliers and the general public
Responsible and Sustainable Practice capabilities	The ability to practise within regulatory/ethical/safety frameworks
Research and Information Management capabilities	Ability to remain informed about herbal medicine and advances in knowledge and apply it in clinical practice where appropriate

that has been outlined. Following this, the overall capability was separated into four critical dimensions that were highlighted as particularly important through a review of literature, professional association documents and dialogue with professional stakeholders and with academics on the programme development team. These capability dimensions were named as: (1) technical capabilities, (2) communication capabilities, (3) responsible and sustainable practice capabilities, and (4) research and information management capabilities. These might be considered to be dimensions of any form of professional practice. In order to make the profile of capability specific to the practice of Chinese medicine, under each of the four dimensions of capabilities, specific capabilities were identified. An example is provided in Table 16.1. Specific *underpinning skills and abilities* that would need to be developed in order to achieve these dimensions of capability were then identified and underlying these, the necessary *enabling knowledge*. This level of specification grounded the broad dimensions within the specific practice context. An example is provided in Table 16.2.

What resulted from this endeavour was a profile or map of capability at a quite detailed level. In developing the overall curriculum model and

Table 16.2. Example of construction of a capability map.

Technical capabilities	Underpinning skills and abilities	Enabling knowledge
The ability to apply knowledge of Chinese medicine principles and diagnosis skills in diagnosis of disease	• Ability to understand the principles of Chinese medicine (theoretical framework) • Skill in taking a case history according to both Chinese and western medicine principles • Skill in performing the four diagnostic techniques of Chinese medicine • Ability to synthesize information about the patient according to Chinese medicine theory	• Knowledge of the philosophies, principles of Chinese medicine including theoretical framework, aetiology, pathogenesis • Knowledge of Chinese medicine terminology • Knowledge of the four diagnostic techniques and data interpretation

the specification for each of the courses that make up the programme, the capability profile was mapped over various potential designs until one was identified that met the needs of a capability approach and fitted within institutional constraints.

Once the capability map for the curriculum had been developed, specific individual courses were identified that needed to be provided within the overall programme in order to achieve the capabilities identified. The capability map was mapped over individual courses. This will be discussed in the next section.

Tables 16.1 and 16.2 thus illustrate stages in the developmental process. Table 16.1 sets out four dimensions of capability identified as essential to the development of the overall, integrative capability and provides an example of each. Table 16.2 illustrates how the capability map was developed using a technical dimension capability as an example.

16.4.1 *Development and integration of specific courses within the overall programme*

Once a conceptual model for the curriculum had been developed based on the principles described above, specific individual courses (subjects) were identified that needed to be provided within the overall programme in order to achieve the capabilities (identified in the capability map). The capabilities, skills and abilities and enabling knowledge were then mapped over individual courses so that a coherent, comprehensive and integrated learning and assessment experience resulted.

Learning outcomes for individual courses then related to these skills and abilities and enabling knowledge that needed to be developed within the course.

In keeping with an integrative approach to curriculum development, specific capabilities and/or skills and abilities were developed concurrently within different courses and/or built on capabilities and/or skills and abilities developed in chronologically earlier courses. In this way, different courses were either reinforcing learning of skills and abilities learned in other courses or developing such skills and abilities further and ultimately, facilitating the learning of capabilities that require the contribution of many underlying skills and abilities to be realised.

For each course, specific capability dimensions were identified as being introduced and/or emphasised. These are documented in the Reference Course Guides for individual courses that provide specifications for the delivery of each course (discussed in the following section). For example, the course "Fundamentals in Chinese Medicine" *emphasises* development of Technical capabilities, particularly the principles that guide Chinese medicine, practical skills in diagnosis and ability to synthesise information according to Chinese medicine theory. It also *introduces* the following dimensions of capabilities:

- Communication capabilities — introduces the ability to communicate bilaterally with an emphasis on communicating diagnoses with the patient
- Responsible and Sustainable Practice capabilities — introduces the regulatory and ethical frameworks and ability to continue to learn
- Research and Information Management capabilities — introduces the concept of evidence-based practice and ability to conduct a literature search

Within individual courses, the level to which each ability and skill (contributing to a specific capability) would be developed was also specified as one of three levels. *Foundation level* describes a basic level of capability, *Intermediate level* describes a higher level of capability than that of Foundation level but one which lacks the required practical experience to be professionally competent, and *Professional level* describes a level sufficient to be professionally competent. Courses in the first year developed capabilities at a foundation or intermediate level, and subsequent courses built on these capabilities developing them to the more sophisticated professional level by the end of the programme. In this way, the curriculum model facilitated development of progressively more sophisticated levels of ability within all dimensions of the overall practice capability.

A range of courses within the programme build towards the overall integrative, real life practice capability. The clinical courses incorporated simulations, role-plays and critical analysis of practice situations and assessment was aligned to real life learning context by the use of major, holistic practice assessments with reflective components managed through a learning log or portfolio. Assessment incorporated practical, performative assessment components with extensive use of peer and self assessments that bring the variation in experience into explicit focus.

16.4.2 *Documenting and communicating requirements for individual courses*

A new concept was utilised as a means of documenting and communicating the requirements for individual courses within the programme so that the desired capability outcome might be achieved. These documents were named *Reference Course Guides* and provided a performance specification for the detailed design of courses that needed to be developed and taught within the programme. They described the capabilities the specific course were required to introduce or emphasise, and the necessary skills and abilities (and underpinning enabling knowledge) that made up the course content and needed to be developed and assessed within it. Within the Reference Course Guides, these were further detailed as learning outcomes and accompanied by suggestions concerning the types of learning experiences and assessment strategies that would facilitate the desired development of capability.

Table 16.3. Example of a capability pathway for the course Chinese Materia Medica and Formulae 2.

(1) The **Technical capabilities** (developed in Chinese Materia Medica and Formulae 2) will build on those developed in:

- Chinese Materia Medica and Formulae 1
- Chinese Medicine Research 1
- Fundamentals of Chinese Medicine

and will be *further developed* in:

- Classic Literature in Chinese Medicine
- Clinical Chinese Medicine 1 to 4
- Pharmacology & Toxicology 1 & 2
- Medicinal Chemistry and Botany
- Chinese Medicine Research 2

(2) The **Communication capabilities** (developed in Chinese Materia Medica and Formulae 2) will build on those learnt in Chinese Materia Medica and Formulae 1 and extended in Clinical Chinese Medicine 1 to 4.

(3) The **Responsible and Sustainable Practice capabilities** will build on those developed in Chinese Materia Medica and Formulae 1 and be extended in Clinical Chinese Medicine 1 to 4.

(4) The **Research and Information management capabilities** (particularly those relating to Evidence-Based practice) will build on those developed in Chinese Materia Medica and Formulae 1 and Chinese Medicine Research 1 and will be *threaded through* all of the clinical courses (including Clinical Chinese Medicine 1 to 4).

The level that each specific ability and skill contributing to a specific capability would be developed to in each course was specified in the Reference Course Guides: foundation, intermediate or professional levels.

The Reference Course Guides also document "Capability pathways" that articulate how the capabilities in individual courses are linked between courses, either through building on previous courses or concurrent or further development within other courses. In this way, the dimensions of capabilities are integrated and reinforced and build on each other. The following example in Table 16.3 illustrates this.

16.4.3 *Integration of Chinese and western medicine*

Integration of Chinese and western medicine was a feature of the curriculum. The grounding of the programme in the context of practice, within a western health care setting that supports predominantly western medicine, is clearly an example of such integration. The integration of Chinese and western medicines occurred within the four dimensions of capabilities identified: technical, communication, responsible and sustainable practice, and research and information management capabilities.

Integration also occurred at each of the next two levels within the capability map: at the level of specific underlying skills and abilities and enabling knowledge. As part of the grounding of the programme within a professional context, ethics and regulatory frameworks were also threaded throughout many of the courses, in particular the clinical courses. The regulatory frameworks stem directly from the western health care system that has developed around western medicine. In terms of integration of knowledge from both systems of medicine about health, disease (including aetiology and pathogenesis), diagnosis and treatment, this was specified within the technical capability dimension and applied at the course level,

Table 16.4. Examples of integration of Chinese and western medicine within the four dimensions of capability.

Dimension of capability	Example of specific capability
Technical capabilities	Ability to diagnose and differentiate diseases/disorders of internal medicine, gynaecology, paediatrics, ENT and ophthalmology, traumatology and dermatology, according to both western and Chinese medicine principles and techniques and formulate an appropriate Chinese herbal formula
Communication capabilities	Ability to refer to medical and other allied health professionals
Responsible and sustainable practice capabilities	The ability to practise within regulatory/ethical/safety frameworks
Research and information management capabilities	Ability to critically review research publications relevant to Chinese medicine

in particular within the clinical courses. Finally, the evidence-based approach born out of western medicine and that increasingly guides clinical practice has been applied to the understanding of Chinese medicine throughout the programme and is discussed in the following section.

Table 16.4 sets out an example of integration of Chinese and western medicine at the capability level.

16.4.4 *Integration of evidence-based approaches in the curriculum*

The importance of an evidence-based approach to the study, practice and research of Chinese medicine was explicit in the identification of the **Research and Information Management capability** dimension as one of the four dimensions of the overall capability. A number of relevant capabilities were then identified under this heading along with skills and abilities that needed to be developed in order to achieve the capabilities, and the enabling knowledge that underpins the skills and abilities. Research and Information Management capabilities were then mapped over individual courses within the programme.

In order to equip practitioners with the capabilities to continue lifelong learning and develop an evidence-based approach to the practice and study of Chinese medicine, two specific research courses were developed. The first of these, Chinese Medicine Research 1, is introduced in Year 1 of the programme and the second, Chinese Medicine Research 2, is introduced in Year 3 and builds on the skills learned in the first course.

Evidence-based approaches including relevant capabilities developed in the Research courses are threaded throughout the programme. For example, many of the courses draw on the information-searching and critical analysis abilities developed in the initial course, Chinese Medicine Research 1. Individual clinical courses are expected to include reference to contemporary literature and research into the different diseases covered in each course including the evidence base for particular treatment approaches. Chinese Medicine Research 2 addresses real world research issues and evidence-based clinical practice, contributing towards an overall integrative focus of the programme.

An example of one of the capabilities identified within the Research and Information management capability dimension is set out in Table 16.5 along with examples of underpinning skills and abilities and enabling knowledge.

Table 16.5. Example of a specific capability within the *Research and Information Management Capability* dimension.

Specific capability	Underpinning skills and abilities include:	Enabling knowledge include (but are not limited to):
The ability to critically review research publications relevant to Chinese medicine	• The ability to continue professional development and education • Skills in interpreting bio-statistics and research methodology • Skills in evaluating research findings • The ability to understand the fundamental elements of design and conduct of laboratory and clinical trials that evaluate safety, quality, and efficacy of Chinese herbal medicines	• Knowledge of what is evidence-based practice • Knowledge of key Chinese medicine, western medical/ biomedical and complementary medicine resources including electronic and printed material • Knowledge of the strategies for making a search for information and literature • Appreciation of the journal refereeing process and publication bias • Awareness of opportunities for continuing education including requirements of professional and registering bodies • Understanding of the unique nature of complementary medicine including Chinese medicine and the need for *appropriate* research methodology that tests the practice appropriately • Knowledge of research tools including biostatistics and research methodology

16.5 Conclusion

RMIT University has taken an approach to the development of a Chinese medicine curriculum that is both innovative and integrative. It integrates Chinese and western medicine in a number of ways. These include specifically the grounding of the programme firmly within the context of practice within a western health care setting, including the inter-leaving of ethics and regulatory frameworks throughout the programme, presentation of medical knowledge from both Chinese and western medicine viewpoints and threading through the programme of an evidence-based approach to the study, practice and research of Chinese medicine. It is integrative in terms of the actual design of the curriculum and this integrative theme is carried through from the level of overall programme design to the creation of Reference Course Guides that guide the detailed design of individual courses within the programme. It is innovative due to all of these reasons and also because of its vision to provide graduates with the capabilities to practice professionally within a rapidly changing health care system.

References

A C Nielson Research Services (2000) *Employer Satisfaction with Graduate Skills: Research Report.* Evaluations and Investigations Programme: Higher Education Division, DETYA.

Business/Higher Education Round Table (BHERT) (2003) *Generic Skills and Higher Education.*

Bensky, D. and Gamble, A. (1993) *Chinese Herbal Medicine Materia Medica*, Eastland Press, Seattle, Washington.

Bowden, J., Hart, G., King, B., Trigwell, K. and Watts, O. (2000) *Generic Capabilities of ATN University Graduates.* Australian Technology Network Teaching and Learning Committee, Final Report to DETYA.

Bowden, J. and Marton, F. (1998) *The University of Learning: Beyond Quality and Competence in Higher Education*, Kogan Page, London.

Cai, J., Chao, G., Chen, D., Chen, X., Cheng, X., *et al.* (1995) *Advanced Textbook on Traditional Chinese Medicine and Pharmacology*, Vol. 1, New World Press, Beijing, China.

Cheng, X. (ed.) (1987) *Chinese Acupuncture and Moxibustion*, Foreign Languages Press, Beijing, China.

Easthope, G., Beilby, J. and Tranter B. (1998) Acupuncture in Australian general practice: practitioners characteristics. *Med. J. Aust.* **169**, 197–200.

Harvey, L. (2000) Graduate employability. In: *Proceedings of the 12th International Conference on Assessing Quality in Higher Education*, Melbourne.

Industry Taskforce on Leadership and Management Skills (Karpin Report) (1995) *Enterprising Nation: Renewing Australia's Managers to Meet the Challenges of the Asia-Pacific Century.* Australia Government Publishing Service, Canberra.

Richardson, J. (2002) Evidence-based complementary medicine: rigor, relevance and the swampy lowlands. *J. Altern. Complement. Med.* **8**(2), 221–223.

Rosenberg, W. (2001) Evidence-based gastroenterology and hepatology. Available at: http://www.library.utoronto.ca/medicine/cbm/syllabi/gas/print/intro.htm [cited 18 March 2004].

Sackett, D.L., Rosenberg, W.M.C., Muir Gray, J.A., Haynes, R.B. and Scott Richardson, W. (1996) Evidence-based medicine: what it is and what it isn't. Available at http://www.cebm.net/ebm_is_isnt.asp [cited 18 March 2004].

Stephenson, J. (1995) Developing the autonomous learner — a capability approach. In: *Proceedings from the 2nd National Information Literacy Conference*, Adelaide.

Tang, J.L. and Wong, T.M. (1998) The need to evaluate the clinical effectiveness of traditional Chinese medicine. *Hong Kong Med. J.* **4**, 208–210.

Index